THE SEITAI METHOD

THE SEITAI METHOD

A Holistic Approach to Staying Healthy through Stretching
and Body Alignment—A Self-Treatment Guide

KUNIAKI IMOTO, Ph.D.

Translated by
William Fedchuk and Makoto Shimamine

KODANSHA INTERNATIONAL
Tokyo · New York · London

NOTE FROM THE PUBLISHER: Those with health problems are advised to seek the guidance of a qualified medical or psychological professional before implementing any of the approaches presented in this book. It is essential that any readers who have any reason to suspect serious illness in themselves or their family members seek appropriate medical, nutritional, or psychological advice promptly. Neither this nor any other health-related book should be used as a substitute for qualified care or treatment. Pregnant women, women in a postnatal period, and individuals in a post-operative period, in particular, should be careful when performing any exercise in this book.

Pregnant women as well as women in a postnatal period, should not perform the following exercises:

Foot bath (p. 38)
Exercise for strained back (B) (p. 44)
V-shape hip joint exercise (p. 46)
Lifting the occipital region using both hands (p. 95)
Exercise for overeating (p. 97)
Exercise to relieve constipation (p. 98)
Pelvic exercise (pp. 100–101)
Exercise for L5 (p. 103)
Iliac bone exercise (pp. 123–125)
Lower back exercise (pp. 125–127)
Combined exercise (pp. 127–129)
Sacrum exercise (pp. 133–134)
Pubic bone exercise (pp. 135–137)

WEBSITE: www.imoto-seitai.com

Photos: Kyuzo Akashi
Model: Kaori Hirawata

Distributed in the United States by Kodansha America, Inc., and in the United Kingdom and continental Europe by Kodansha Europe Ltd.

Published by Kodansha International Ltd., 17–14 Otowa 1-chome, Bunkyo-ku, Tokyo 112–8652, and Kodansha America, Inc.

First edition, 2004
10 09 08 07 06 05 04 10 9 8 7 6 5 4 3 2 1

www.kodansha-intl.com

CONTENTS

FOREWORD

It has long been recognized that modern medical science has been making 'progress.' Indeed, the discovery of antibiotics, for example, has meant that illnesses caused by bacteria that had once run rampant, such as cholera and tuberculosis, are no longer fatal. Technology, equipment, and methods used in medical examinations and surgical operations have also improved immensely. Such 'progress' has made the early detection and correct treatment of various diseases and symptoms possible.

Progress has undoubtedly been made, yet many diseases that Western medical science is finding difficult to cure thrive around the world—AIDS, cancer, diabetes, various kinds of liver and kidney disease, rheumatism, asthma, allergies, atopic dermatitis, to name just a few. Moreover, new problems have emerged, such as antibiotic-resistant bacteria, against which conventional antibiotics are ineffective.

Many people who may have no specific illness can still suffer from a variety of mental and physical discomforts. Are we simply to assume that these problems will someday be cured by progress made in Western medical science? Those reading this book must seriously consider this or similar questions.

Simply put, the approach of modern Western medical science is one of symptomatic treatment—aimed at suppressing symptoms when they appear, taking some form of supplement when the body is lacking something, and removing a body part when it is diseased. Modern Western medical science is adept at addressing the symptoms, but does not appear to adequately pinpoint the source of the problem.

Can such measures as suppressing a fever, administering hormone medicine, or removing a cancerous growth be considered fundamental medical solutions without first ascertaining the source of the problem?

The human body has the power to restore itself naturally to its normal condition from common illness and injury without external interference. This we call the body's natural healing power. While this natural healing power works unconsciously, various factors that weaken or obstruct its ability to function are revealed to the Seitai practitioner when examining the condition of the body's skeletal frame and muscles.

Seitai is a method that activates the natural healing power of the body by determining the source of a problem and thereafter applying the appropriate Seitai techniques. Seitai combines the essence of hidden techniques of the masters of various healing therapies that existed in Japan at the time of the Second World War. Fearing that their secret techniques would be lost, the masters of various therapies assembled to scrutinize each technique, and to select and preserve only those that were absolutely effective. Seitai developed from the combination and perfection of such techniques. Until then, the so-called "secret" or "esoteric" healing techniques had traditionally been passed down to only a few recipients in Japan and other Asian countries.

I began learning Seitai from my father, a Seitai master, when I was five years old. However, my own techniques have changed significantly from those of the original Seitai, and even those of my father, since I have adopted my own discoveries and ideas into my form of Seitai in accordance with the changes I have witnessed occurring in the human body over the past fifty years. For this reason, I have named my particular Seitai theory and techniques "Imoto Seitai" (hereinafter, Seitai).

I studied Western medical science and other Oriental medicines when I was young and later established a private hospital to realize my dream of fusing Western medical science and Seitai. However, in spite of such exhaustive efforts, I reached the conclusion that Seitai cannot be matched by any other medical discipline.

I have been teaching my Seitai theory and techniques to Japanese and foreign students in order to properly introduce the magnificent teachings of Seitai. This book represents my wholehearted effort to spread some of the knowledge of life and the human body that I have accumulated through my lifelong practice of Seitai.

This book introduces the basic principles of Seitai, original Seitai physical exercises, and the hot moist towel method in detail, supplemented with photographs and illustrations, aiming to provide a precise explanation for the general reader.

It is my sincere hope that more people will explore the superiority of Seitai and, moreover, the excellence and perfection of the power of the human body.

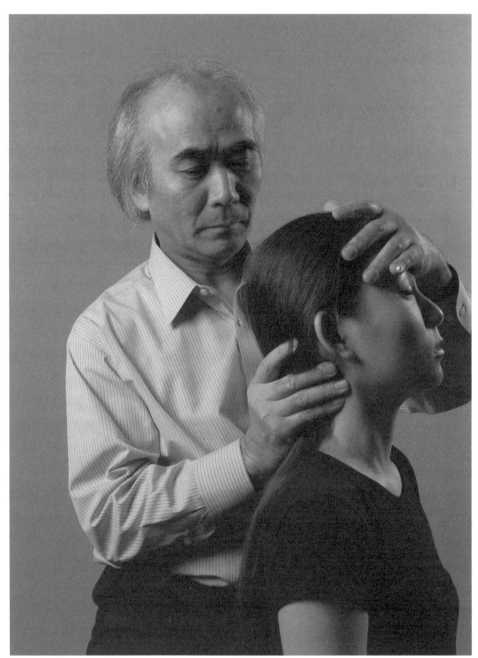

The author checking the condition of the recipient's head and neck.

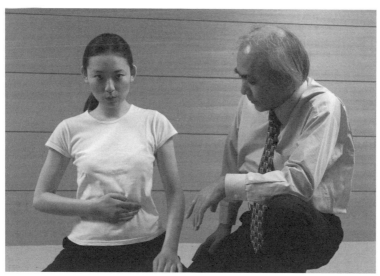

The author consulting with a recipient.

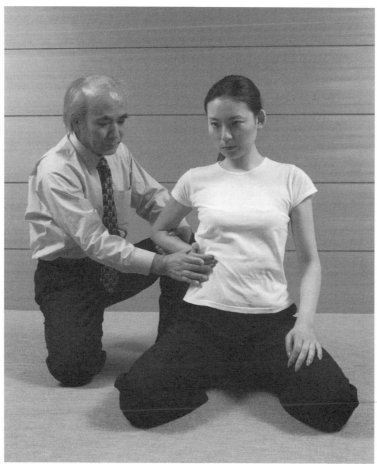

The author administering treatment to the recipient.

Chapter 1

BASIC THEORY OF SEITAI

ILLNESS—Destruction Before Construction

One response to the question "What does it mean to be healthy?" might be, "That's easy! Being healthy means not being sick."

This may seem correct, but is it really true?

Another might say, "I am confident of my health. I haven't caught a single cold during the entire year."

From the Seitai point of view, however, the individual who never catches a cold is not healthy. A body that is properly sensitive to catching a cold under natural conditions is regarded as healthy. In other words, this is the condition of the body we refer to as Seitai—a body in good order. On the contrary, a body that seldom catches a cold is considered to be dull and insensitive. The condition of such a body is the opposite to Seitai and therefore unhealthy.

From the Seitai point of view, the human body becomes sick in order to cure problems that arise in the body. In other words, the body initiates various responses to rid itself of accumulated problems when they exceed the manageable limit for that particular individual. This normal function of the body is generally referred to as "illness" or "disease."

For example, the various symptoms of a cold include fever, headache, cough, runny nose, vomiting, and diarrhea. Generally, such symptoms of "illness" are considered undesirable or unhealthy. Seitai, however, regards these symptoms as the body's natural response to restore itself to its original condition.

When constructing a new building on an existing building site, it is necessary to demolish the old building and remove the rubble from the area. In a similar way, the body destroys the part that becomes too old, that is no longer useful, or that is not in proper working order, and excretes it. Destruction and excretion completed, the construction process begins. The various symptoms of a cold comprise the process of such destruction and excretion, and once construction is completed, the refreshed body is eradicated of the previous accumulated problems and is left feeling invigorated.

A Seitai body is highly sensitive and responds to the subtlest problems, regardless of whether the source of the problem is external or internal, and attempts to cure itself. Therefore, a highly sensitive individual might seem vulnerable to illness, but the symptoms of the illness are light and easily alleviated, since the problem remains small. For instance, a Seitai body can shake off a cold with just a few sneezes.

Meanwhile, a body that is dull and not sufficiently sensitive fails to initiate a curative response until the problem grows considerably. Such a body seems resistant to sickness, but once it develops illness, the body's response is intense and prolonged owing to the accumulation of problems. If the degree of the response exceeds the limit of physical endurance, the illness may become fatal in some cases.

Recently, the concept of the "natural healing power" of the body has been attracting attention. It seems that people have grown accustomed to the term and think they understand it adequately. However, while the term is generally recognized as the power to recover from illness and injury, it is important to remember that becoming ill also comprises a vital part of the natural healing power. Hence, developing an illness indicates that the individual has already moved one step toward recovering to his or her original and healthy physical condition.

THE TRUE NATURE OF THE BODY FROM THE SEITAI PERSPECTIVE

Tension and relaxation

The human body and mind experience varying degrees of tension and relaxation on a daily basis. In the case of breathing, for example, the body tenses when inhaling and relaxes when exhaling. Most daytime activities are tension-related and at night-time, sleep allows the body to relax. This cycle can also be viewed as an alternation between concentration and dispersion.

Moreover, even longer cycles of tension and relaxation are repeated over a week, a month, three months, half a year, one year, three years, and longer. In this overall cycle of time, death can be seen as the final resting period for the body.

Another important cycle of body change coincides with the movement from one season to another, as the body adapts to changes in such climatic factors as temperature and humidity.

If the body is not properly exerted, it will become increasingly difficult for it to fully relax. People leading active lives during the day enjoy a good night's rest. Conversely, people who are unable to sleep well suffer from sluggishness and decreased performance during the active part of their day.

In order to enjoy life with vitality, it is important to keep a healthy balance regarding the cycle of tension and relaxation. In modern society, more and more people are losing this balance.

If the body remains relaxed and flexible, one can easily maintain this balance without effort. A constantly stiff body cannot tolerate further tension, nor can it relax easily.

The problem of the human body in modern society

There are several reasons why the body has become stiff in modern society. Most notably, perhaps, is the distortion of the body frame due to the downward shift of the pelvis.

The spinal column, the core vertical axis of the body, and the lumbar and the pelvis, supporting the upper half of the body, are of utmost importance for human beings, who stand upright, to function properly.

A flexible spinal column naturally forms an elongated "S" shape. Likewise, the pelvis shifts up and the lumbar region arches inward. In such a condition, the upper half of the body is properly supported by the pelvis, which is supported by the legs. No discomfort or feeling of imbalance is experienced if one maintains this ideal posture.

The shifting of the pelvis downward for whatever reason can adversely affect the scapula, causing them to spread out laterally and shift down. This condition can cause such symptoms as heart and lung trouble, stiff shoulders, and neck pain. The lowering of the scapula also affects the ribs and stiffens the intercostals, which can also be the source of various problems and diseases.

The shifting of the scapula can also produce the effect of lowering the occipital area, depriving the cervical vertebrae of flexibility. Various problems might also arise in the eyes, ears, nose, teeth, and the brain, leading to an inability to concentrate.

The extent to which the pelvis lowers on the left or right sides can also influence how the upper half of the body is affected. The correct position of the pelvis is vital in dispersing the force concentrated along the central vertical axis and any lowering of the pelvis can therefore lead to abnormalities in the body. If the force in the body disperses from the central vertical axis, the body starts to tense unnaturally in an effort to maintain balance. This is the reason the body stiffens.

Aside from external physical causes, such as bruising, the lowering of the pelvis can be attributed to the following reasons:

(a) Overwork
(b) Excessive stress
(c) Excessive physical exercise
(d) Overeating
(e) Incorrect post-natal care

As the latter topic is all but ignored by Western medical science, the Seitai viewpoint is as follows.

After child delivery, the pelvis closes gradually, alternating between the left and right sides in eight–hour periods. It takes 7–10 weeks for the pelvis to fully recover to its original position. If any excessive burden is placed on the pelvis and its related body parts during this process, the pelvis ceases to close properly and remains distorted. As this condition cannot be adjusted easily, standing soon after the delivery must be avoided at all cost, as must any activity that would stimulate an area of the body related to the pelvis. Shampooing the hair, for instance, would affect the occipital region, which is related to the pelvis. For more information, please contact Imoto Seitai by E-mail.

Individuals in modern society perspire less frequently

Nowadays, the use of air conditioning in most buildings reduces the opportunity to perspire naturally. If sweat breaks out while outdoors, the mechanism is suppressed and the body cools down when entering an air-conditioned environment. Perspiring adjusts the body's temperature and aids metabolism by excreting body waste, such as lactic acid. By restricting the perspiration process, body waste builds up inside the body, resulting in stiffness.

Moreover, a close relationship exists between perspiration and other metabolic functions. A body with a poor ability to perspire will not be able to maintain a constant body temperature, possibly leading to such symptoms as hypothermia. Furthermore, the body will not effectively be able to induce a fever and regenerate, which will result in further stiffening.

Symptoms must not be suppressed with medicine

If the natural function of the body to recover to its normal condition is identified as a disease and this process is suppressed with medicine, the recovery process is interrupted and the body stiffens. In other words, the abnormality remains in the body.

For more information concerning this topic, please refer to the section titled "Illness—Destruction Before Construction (p. 12)."

Seitai makes the most suitable body

In a healthy body, one that is relaxed and flexible, the forces of the muscles and the body frame are concentrated along the central vertical axis of the body (i.e. the spinal column) to keep the body stable and erect. Imagine the appearance of a tired person sitting in a chair as an example of the body in a bad condition. As the posture indicates, the force in the body flows away from the central axis. This causes partial stiffness in the body, which is the source of various abnormalities.

Reconcentrating the force toward the central vertical axis recovers flexibility in the body and eliminates the abnormalities. Manipulating and adjusting just one or a few vital points in the recipient's body is sufficient to redirect the flow of force toward the central vertical axis.

In Seitai, disease names have no relevance. The body is designed to revert to its original condition, irrespective of the name of a symptom or disease. By provoking the sensibility of the recipient, Seitai techniques stimulate the body to recognize an abnormality and lead it to its normal condition.

The creation of Seitai Exercises, Hot Bathing Methods, and the hot moist towel method introduced in this book is based on the aforementioned theoretical background. Through my many years of experience guiding people with Seitai, I have witnessed the extraordinary effects of these techniques countless times.

RESPECT FOR LIFE

Life, which we experience only once, is precious. Looking back on my years of experience of life associated with Seitai, I myself cannot but feel wonder and reverence for the sublimity of life.

The fundamental concept in the basic ideology of Imoto Seitai, of importance to all individuals, is how one expresses gratitude for this magnificent life.

A life is not like a machine. Life varies individually and changes continuously. A Seitai practitioner must be sensitive to all the subtle differences and changes in the individual body. Therefore, a Seitai treatment is not at all similar to massaging a recipient's body in accordance with a prescribed manual.

The Seitai practitioner approaches the recipient's life with complete devotion, making every effort to guide that life in the direction that is most appropriate for the individual's unique constitution. The recipient too is required to have a sincere attitude to accept the guidance.

Such pure interaction between practitioner and recipient generates the mutual enhancement of KI—the body's vital energy—and makes Seitai treatment possible.

The relationship between the Seitai practitioner and the recipient is unlike any other. The closest comparison might be that of a teacher and a student. The Seitai practitioner must take the role of leading the recipient to a higher level of well-being, and must possess and maintain superior skill to lead the recipient appropriately.

The role of the Seitai practitioner is not to give recipients what they *want*, but to guide them to recognize what they actually *need*. This is achieved by the practitioner's ability to precisely assess the recipient's physical, mental, and emotional states of health.

Also, because of its high degree of earnestness, Seitai places emphasis on proper conduct. An example of such conduct is observed at the start of the Seitai treatment, with a mutual bow between the practitioner and the recipient, as an expression of respect for one another's lives. Observing proper conduct from the heart is the first step toward giving full respect to life.

WHAT IS "KI?"

Countless studies have been performed and many books have been written on the subject of KI, especially in the East. Japan also has a long history of the application of KI to various fields, such as medicine, martial arts, etc. So-called "scientific research" about KI is abundant, and various theories have been published concerning the true nature of KI. Meanwhile, focusing on the introduction of Imoto Seitai, I cannot proceed further without expressing my theories concerning KI, which are based on my experience of dedicated observation of living human bodies for more than 50 years.

KI is LIFE itself

KI *flows* and *circulates* in all living things. It is something that one *feels* in a living body. A human body is made of cells. If cells were to divide repeatedly into the smallest possible unit, the one thing that would remain after all else is removed is KI.

A cell is a concentration of KI. When cells gather and create a body, LIFE resides in the body. Each cell is filled with KI. Through the function of KI, cells regenerate and LIFE is maintained. In other words, KI is that very phenomenon we have called a "soul" since long ago. I have reached this conclusion concerning KI over many years of sincere observation of living human bodies.

KI is something that flows and circulates

Infants are full of vital energy and their bodies are warm and flexible. A dead body is cold and stiff. An area of the body that harnesses KI, on the other hand, is warm and flexible; the KI flows. Needless to say, a body without KI is lifeless, but even an area of the body in which KI does not flow unrestricted can be described as 'partially dead.'

When cancer cells, for instance, destroy normal cells and regeneration has ceased, the area is cold and stiff. In such areas, I feel that the flow of KI has become stagnant.

An area where KI is weak causes various discomforts and problems in the body. Therefore, if KI is attracted to and intensified in such specific areas, the entire body reverts to a healthy condition. The ultimate aim of the various techniques of Seitai is nothing other than to enhance the KI of recipients.

KI is in Everyone

KI is not something that can be transferred from one person to another. KI exists naturally in everyone's body. Though it seems that members of certain groups concerned with the practice of KI maintain that they have the ability to transfer their own KI into a recipient's body, I do not adopt such a position. If KI does not exist in the recipient's body, all efforts by another to instill KI into that body are entirely futile. Even Seitai practitioners are restricted by what they are able to do with their own KI, and that is nothing other than to lead recipients to recognize obstructions of the flow of KI in their bodies, and to help them regain their natural flow of KI by means of their own strength.

KI is Something to FEEL

When shaking hands, embracing another person, seeing the appearance of a friend or listening to the voices of others, one naturally has a sense that others are *alive*. This is also a way of *feeling* the KI of others.

Another example of the sensation of KI is when a loving couple holds hands. As well as their hands, their entire bodies become warm, but this warming effect cannot be attributed to the temperature of the hands. When we touch the hand of a complete stranger, the sensation is completely different. In such a manner, we naturally feel and fully utilize KI in daily life without giving it any thought.

THE BACKBONE INFLUENCES THE WHOLE BODY

The human body is supported by the spinal column, or backbone. The spinal column is comprised of a series of 24 articulated bones called vertebrae. In descending order along the spinal column, the vertebrae are grouped into four sections—cervical vertebrae (7 vertebrae), thoracic vertebrae (12 vertebrae), lumbar vertebrae (5 vertebrae), and sacrum vertebrae (5 fused vertebrae). The ability of the vertebrae to move freely and independently enables the various complex and dynamic movements of the body, such as bending, twisting, and stretching.

As well as providing the chief support for the body and functioning as the central axis of the body's movement, the spinal column encases the spinal cord. The brain and spinal cord make up the central nervous system and a peripheral nervous system branches out from the spinal cord to all other parts of the body. For this reason, an injury to the spinal column usually results in a serious disability.

Even if the spinal column does not appear to be injured, various abnormalities manifest in the body as vertebrae lose flexibility, thereby obstructing nerve transmission to the related organs.

Likewise, the irregular function of an organ is indicated by the stiffening of the related vertebra(e).

In Seitai, a practitioner first manually examines the condition of each vertebra and then manipulates the specific vertebra or selected points on the muscles on either side of the vertebra to induce a direct effect on the muscle, as well as an indirect effect on the related vertebra(e) and body part.

The relationship between each vertebra and the related internal organs/system in Seitai is indicated on the following page. (The vertebrae are numbered in descending order starting at 1. For the purpose of brevity, upper case letters C, T, L, and S are used throughout this text to denote the cervical, thoracic, lumbar, and sacrum vertebrae, respectively.)

Cervical vertebrae (7 vertebrae)

C1, C2	Blood circulation in the head
C3	Nasal mucous membrane
C4	Ears
C5, C6	Throat
C7	Increase in vagus nerve tension

Thoracic vertebrae (12 vertebrae)

T1, T2	Blood circulation in the trachea mucous membrane
T2	Stomach and liver
T3	Lungs
T4	Esophagus, liver, lungs, and heart
T5	Contraction of the cardia
T6	Lesser visceral nerves, vascular movement of the stomach
T7	Spleen, digestive organs
T8	Pancreas, spleen, and pleura
T9	Liver, gall bladder, and expansion of the aorta
T10	Kidneys, eyesight
T8, T9, T10	Bloating of the stomach
T11, T12	Small intestine, ovaries, and testicles

Lumbar vertebrae (5 vertebrae)

L1	Sexual organs, mental perception, and head
L1, L2	Sexual organs
L2	Large intestine and appendix
L3	Sexual organs, blood circulation, kidneys
L4	Ovaries and testicles
L5	Bladder

Sacrum (5 fused vertebrae)

S1, S2	Sexual organs
S2	Early detection of pregnancy
S4	Anus, bladder, and sphincter
S4, S5	Sphincter of gluteal region

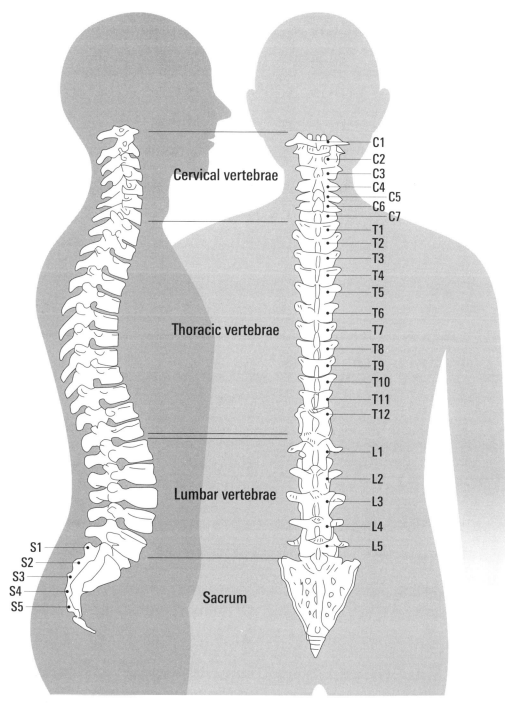

Cervical vertebrae

Thoracic vertebrae

Lumbar vertebrae

Sacrum

C1
C2
C3
C4
C5
C6
C7
T1
T2
T3
T4
T5
T6
T7
T8
T9
T10
T11
T12
L1
L2
L3
L4
L5

S1
S2
S3
S4
S5

The 24 vertebrae and 5 fused vertebrae of the sacrum.

Chapter 2

ASSESS THE BODY WITH 7 POSTURES

It is possible to assess the condition of the body with the following seven simple postures and movements.

TURNING THE NECK

The source of neck trouble is seldom found in the neck itself, but more often in three body parts connected to the neck—the chest, the back, and the arms. Therefore, manipulating the neck itself cannot be a fundamental solution for neck trouble, and such manipulation may cause a more serious problem. Careful attention is necessary.

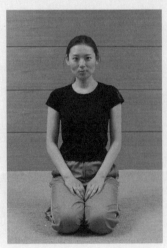

Sit down.

1. Difficulty looking up

A) STIFFNESS IN C7 AND T1

Some stiffness appears in the joint between the last cervical (C7) and first thoracic (T1) vertebrae. The joint between C7 and T1 is affected and stiffens as a result of overuse of the arms and hands, such as would occur when nursing a patient or the elderly, or through prolonged use of a personal computer.

B) TIRED LUMBAR AREA

When the lumbar area drops down, the neck stiffens, and turning

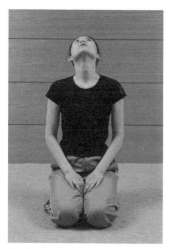

Look up.

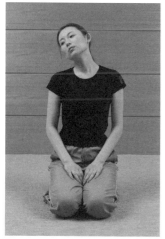

Turn the head left or right.

the neck becomes difficult. The causes of the downward shift of the lumbar are various, such as physical fatigue, mental stress, excessive exercising, overeating, a blow to the lumbar region, and incorrect post-natal care.

C) POOR CIRCULATION OF BODY FLUID

As the symptoms of arteriosclerosis (abnormal thickening and hardening of arterial walls with resulting loss of elasticity) in the body progress, the neck becomes stiff and difficult to turn.

2. Difficulty turning the head left or right

When the muscles on one side of the neck stiffen, this more often indicates a problem in the arm or lung on the same side of the body than trouble in the neck itself. Muscle stiffness in the neck is sometimes an expression of a problem in the heart (left side of neck), kidneys (left and right), stomach (left side), the liver (right side, generally attributed to regular use of medicines, mental stress, and overeating), and gynecological problems (left side). However, when an individual maintains body balance by slightly twisting the body, the source of the trouble in the neck sometimes arises from the opposite side of the body.

3. Difficulty turning the head and neck separately; attempting to move the head only, the neck turns together from the base

The entire neck, especially the upper part, stiffens. Mental fatigue affects the occiput (back of the head) and eventually the neck.

4. Shrugging the shoulders eases turning of the neck

The muscles from the chest up to the neck become stiff when the effect of the downward shift of the ribs reaches the collarbones. Raising the shoulders loosens the stiffness and eases turning of the neck. The main causes of the downward shift of the ribs are lung and heart problems, arm fatigue, or a disorder of the pelvis or pelvic organs.

RAISING THE ARMS OVERHEAD WHILE LYING ON THE BACK

Normally, the left and right arms are raised with equal ease and strength. Each of the raised arms should be straight and touching each ear. The appearance of this pose, as outlined in the following points, informs us of various bodily conditions.

1. Arms bend at the elbows even while trying to stretch the arms straight

The arms bend at the elbows when there is stiffness in the chest or a problem in the arm muscles. The main cause of the stiffness is arm muscle fatigue. If the stiffness is not treated, the wrists stiffen next.

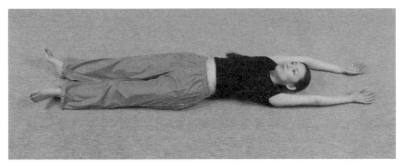

Raise the arms overhead while lying on the back.

2. Difference in the degree of bending of the left and right arms

The arm with the stiffer elbow is more bent. Usually, stiffening begins in the arm with the dominant hand. Thereafter, the opposite arm, which compensates for the weakened dominant arm, also stiffens.

3. The gap between the raised arms and the ears is noticeably wide and differs on each side

The gap between the raised arms and the ears increases when the shoulder blades shift laterally to the outside, owing to fatigue of the entire body or a problem of the respiratory system. The side of the body with the larger gap has an abnormality; in the lung, for instance.

4. Arms can only be raised halfway above the head

With the arms held at the maximum achievable height, imagine drawing a line between the arm and the shoulder blade. An abnormality is found on the outside edge of the shoulder blade at the point where the line meets the shoulder blade. Moreover, the source of the stiffness is determined by tracing the flow of force to the spinal column.

SITTING ON THE FLOOR WITH LEGS EXTENDED FORWARD

When the spinal column is flexible and maintains a normal curve, the center of gravity in the body adjusts easily. The posture is held without effort and the upper body remains fully erect.

1. The posture is unstable unless the legs are opened widely

If it is necessary to open the legs widely to maintain stability, the upper chest is stiff and stiffness is moving into the lumbar area. When the pelvis shifts down, the force concentrated along the body's central vertical axis starts to disperse from the legs. The posture is more easily held by opening the legs widely. As the lumbar increasingly stiffens, the width between the legs widens.

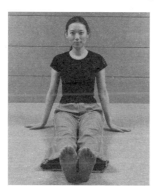 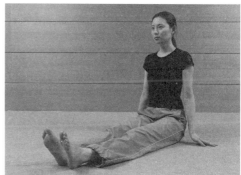

Sit on the floor with legs extended forward.

2. Supporting the body with the arms and hands or rounded back

The center of gravity in the body moves to the back side of the body owing to stiffening of the lumbar. The arms, with hands placed slightly behind the hips, or a rounded upper back, support and maintain the posture.

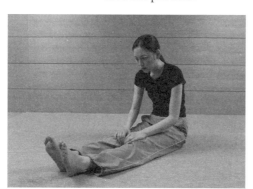 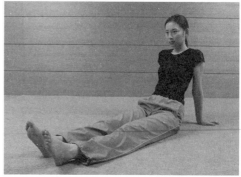

When the body is supported with the arms and hands or a rounded back, the center of gravity in the body moves to the back side of the body.

3. Sit with legs bent and join the soles of the feet

A difference in the height of the knees indicates some trouble in the lumbar, the hip joint, Achilles tendon, ankle, or twisting of the upper chest.

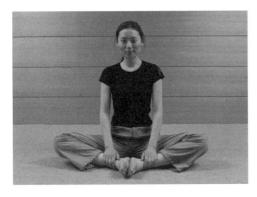

Bend the knees and join the soles of the feet.

STANDING

The posture of a person standing naturally and relaxed reveals various characteristics of the body, since the body is supported on two legs.

1. Feet turned inward

The weight of the upper body is first supported by the pelvis and then transferred to the inside of the knees and down to the large toes. The cause of this position is the downward shifting of the pelvis, or, less frequently, excessive inward curving of the lumbar spine, which raises the hips too high.

2. One foot is in front of the other

This occurs when there is a twist somewhere in the upper body, most commonly at L3. Such individuals are prone to high fevers, serious coughs, and excessive night sweats when they catch a cold. The symptoms persist for a long time.

3. The knees open outward / the width between the feet becomes extremely wide / the feet turn outward

Weight from the upper part of the body passes through the pubis and then down to the outside of the knees. Body balance must be com-

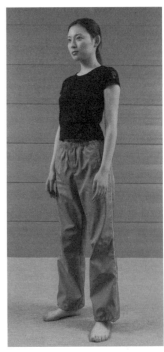

Stand naturally and relaxed.

pensated for when standing upright and, in this case, the inside of the legs are the main support. If the inside ankles are pivotal in adjusting the balance, the legs are bowed. It is easier for such individuals to maintain their posture by widening the distance between the feet or turning the feet outward.

LYING FACE DOWN

Lying face down with arms along the sides of the body relaxes the entire body. Therefore, any partial stiffness in the body is quickly noticeable.

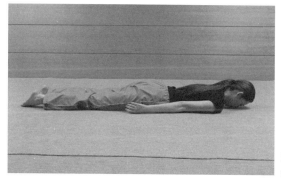

Lie face down with arms along the sides of the body.

1. Unable to lie face down and lift the head

If the body is normally relaxed, the individual feels comfortable, whether the face is turned down, up, left, or right. When difficulty is experienced lying face down, stiffness appears in the joint between C7 and T1. Owing to the stiffness, the area cannot support the head and allow the tension to pass up to the flexible cervical vertebrae. The cause of the stiffness is assumed to be overuse of the arms or fingers. If all the cervical vertebrae stiffen, lying face down is not possible. Such individuals have a higher risk of cerebral hemorrhage.

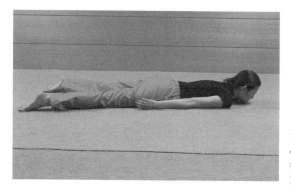

When unable to lie face down and lift the head, stiffness appears in the joint between C7 and T1.

2. The arms are opened widely and cannot rest alongside the body

If the body is properly relaxed, the arms are relaxed and lie naturally alongside the body, and the individual feels comfortable with the palms of the hands facing up or down. In some instances, however, the shoulder blades spread laterally outward when the arms spread excessively away from the body. The cause of this is believed to be a problem in the respiratory system or excessive fatigue. If the lungs are stiff, placing the palms facing the floor relieves pressure on the lungs and increases comfort. If the stiffness in the lungs deteriorates further, the individual has no choice but to place the backs of hands to the floor.

3. The feet are standing

The individual has some mental stress or stiffness in the lumbar or Achilles tendons.

4. The insides of the legs and knees rest on the floor and the feet turn outward

In this position, the pelvis has dropped down. Tension is moving away from the center of the body to the outside of the legs and the body is attempting to again concentrate the tension back to the ilium by using the support of the outside leg muscles and leg joints.

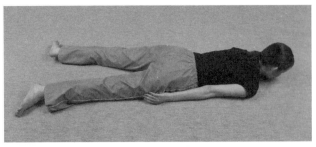

When the insides of the legs and knees rest on the floor and the feet turn outward, the pelvis has dropped down.

5. Legs open beyond the width of the shoulders

The pelvis is abnormally loose. It is assumed that the individual has excessive body fatigue or a constitution that often results in a tumor, such as a myoma, in the organs contained in the pelvis.

LYING ON THE BACK

As all the tension in the legs is released, various problems can be identified by the positioning of the legs. Normally, the feet naturally fall outward and the width of the legs about equals the width of the pelvis.

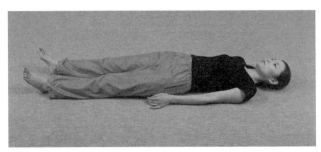

Lie on the back.

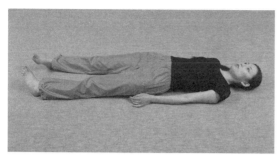

If the feet turn inward, one possible cause is assumed to be atrophy of the pelvis.

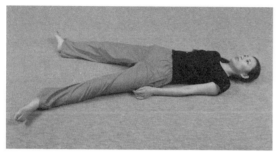

When the feet fall too far outside, the pelvis is abnormally loose and shifts downward.

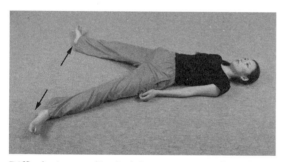

Difficulty in spreading both legs apart at a wide angle can indicate a variety of conditions.

1. Feet turn inward

This position is assumed to be caused by such problems as atrophy of the pelvis, dysfunction of the lungs, and mental stress. It is also an indication of problems in the sexual organs.

2. Feet fall too far outside / both legs excessively wide apart

In both cases, the pelvis is abnormally loose and shifts downward, and excessive fatigue is felt in the lumbar area.

■ SPREADING BOTH LEGS APART
  IN THE SAME POSTURE

(1) One leg is difficult to open.
    Such difficulty is generally an indication of stiffening and downward shift of the lumbar area, hip joint or knee stiffness, kidney malfunction, the aftereffect of a bruise on the pelvis, and problems with blood circulation and nerve transmission on the same side that the difficulty is experienced.

(2) Tension in the thighs and groin.
    If the individual feels too much tension and obstruction in the thighs and groin when trying to open the legs more widely, the force received by the pelvis is transferred to the front of the ilium and then to the pubis. This causes stiffening of the adductor muscles. The causes of the stiffening of the adductor muscles are assumed to be gynecological problems, especially difficult convalescence after a surgical operation, or problems with other pelvic organs, such as the urinary organs or intestines.

LYING FACE DOWN AND ROCKING THE HIPS

1. Difficulty rocking to one side

More resistance is felt moving the hips to the side where the lumbar area or ilium is tense or where there is stiffness in the thighs, or the after-effect of a bruise on the pelvis.

2. Lumbar area moves in unison with the hips.

Normally, lumbar vertebra L2 is the axis for a rocking movement. If L2 is stiff, however, the axis moves up the spine and the entire lumbar area moves in unison. This is related to a problem in the digestive system.

3. Movement of the hips makes the shape of a horizontal figure '8.'

When the movement of the hips creates the shape of a horizontal figure '8,' it indicates that lumbar vertebra L3 is twisted. This is related to a problem with the kidneys.

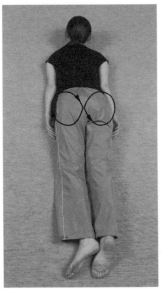 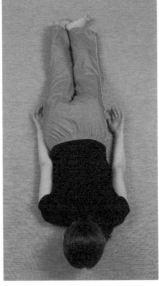

When the movement of the hips creates the shape of a horizontal figure '8,' it indicates that lumbar vertebra L3 is twisted.

Chapter 3

SELF-TREATMENT TECHNIQUES OF IMOTO-SEITAI

The human body is designed to heal an injury and overcome sickness by itself, without any form of external assistance. This is because the body has natural healing power. Fundamentally, Seitai is based on the principle that enhancing the body's natural healing power adjusts and maintains the body in proper order.

Above all, the following four methods of self-treatment are of vital importance within the system of Seitai techniques and adhere to the basic philosophy of Seitai, which is:

EVERYONE SHOULD BE RESPONSIBLE FOR HIS OR HER OWN HEALTH.

1. DOU-KI (leading KI)
2. Seitai Physical Exercises
3. Hot Moist Towel Method
4. Hot Bathing Method

DOU-KI

The DOU-KI method is used to enhance and adjust the KI of recipients by placing a hand on the area of the body experiencing pain or difficulty, and concentrating on the area while imagining inhaling and exhaling from the palm of the hand. DOU-KI can also be done by oneself.

Though this technique may seem unfamiliar, people commonly and naturally place the palm of a hand on an aching point, as when experiencing a headache or stomachache, or when a parent hugs and soothes a crying child by rubbing his or her injury.

The flow of KI is blocked where there is a problem or where the function of a part of the body is failing. Performing DOU-KI to such an area draws the recipient's focus to the area. KI in the recipient's body also concentrates and flows into the area. When the flow of KI is enhanced, the body starts working to adjust itself to its normal condition.

This is the most basic and effective method of DOU-KI. However, it is important to realize that anything that guides KI is DOU-KI. Being in close proximity to, talking to, and looking at someone warmly can have the same effect as DOU-KI.

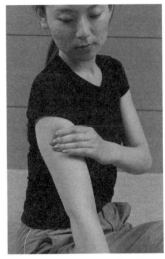

Applying DOU-KI on the Kano-katten (See p. 140)

Moreover, Seitai has developed a method of training called GYOU-KI (austere training of KI) to adjust and enhance KI in your own body.

1. GYOU-KI by holding the hands in a prayer position about 10 cm apart. This is a way of concentrating and enhancing KI in the palms. (See p. 60)

2. GYOU-KI in the spinal column. This method of leading KI through the spinal column steadies the circulation of KI in the body.

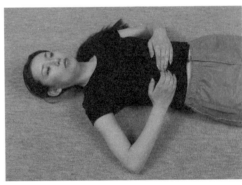

Applying DOU-KI on the Risho-katten (See p. 140)

These two methods of training enhance KI in the body and also purify the individual's physical and mental condition.

SEITAI PHYSICAL EXERCISES

Of the many kinds of physical exercises that exist in the world, Seitai exercises, from the viewpoint of adjusting the body, are the most effective. This is because Seitai exercises fully utilize the characteristics of the body as follows:

1. Partial fatigue

The way a person uses the body differs from one individual to the next depending on the innate characteristics of the body, the habitual way of using the body, the type of job one does, etc. The part of the body that experiences fatigue also differs between individuals. Someone doing deskwork, for example, tends to experience mental and eye fatigue.

Moreover, individuals react differently to external influences, the effect that such influences have in causing mental stress, and subsequently how mental stress manifests as fatigue in the body. The digestive organs are affected in one individual, the respiratory organs in another, and the mental condition in yet another.

In this way, fatigue tends to accumulate in just one area of the body and seldom does the whole body become equally tired.

Fatigue, however, is different from a feeling of tiredness. One may feel mental perception becomes dull when the legs get extremely tired after a long walk. Or, the entire body may feel tired after only using the eyes for a prolonged period. Furthermore, when under extreme mental stress, the whole body might feel tired, even though the body has undergone no physical stress.

In other words, it is the nature of the body to mistake extreme localized fatigue as fatigue throughout the entire body. Even if one feels tired, the body is only tired in one specific area where partial fatigue has accumulated. If such partial fatigue is alleviated, the body recovers significantly and returns to its normal functioning level.

2. "Your" Seitai exercise

The primary characteristic of Seitai exercises is to find the specific point in the body where partial fatigue tends to accumulate, easily creating an abnormality, and to concentrate full attention on that point. Therefore, it is not necessary to move all parts of the body when doing Seitai exercises. The Seitai exercise most beneficial for each person is prescribed individually. Hence, not all people do the same Seitai exercise in the same way.

Seitai prescribes you YOUR OWN unique exercise.

3. Dramatic effects can be achieved in a short time with Seitai exercises

It is not necessary to spend several hours practicing a sport and sweating profusely if the aim is simply to adjust one's physical condition.

One Seitai exercise takes just a few minutes. How can the body be adjusted in such a short time? The reasons are explained in Point 4.

4. Tension and relaxation

A part of the body that functions normally is soft and flexible, and an abnormality, where fatigue accumulates, is often stiff. In some instances, the abnormality can manifest as an overly relaxed area rather like a rubber band that has completely lost its elasticity. In these cases, it is crucial to identify a small, concentrated area of stiffness so that proper treatment can be administered.

Many mainstream relaxation techniques commonly rub and massage a stiff body, as is done when sitting in an electric massaging chair. However, when the body is continuously stimulated in this way, it initially relaxes, but thereafter becomes stiffer and dull to the stimulus as a natural protective reaction. For this reason, over-stimulation of the body, as done by the massaging chair, becomes increasingly unable to adequately satisfy the body and a stronger stimulus is needed to be effective. The degree of stiffness in the body increases proportionally with the rising intensity of the massaging chair.

The body behaves according to the principle that something that endures maximum tension then reverts to maximum relaxation. The most effective way to relax the stiff part of the body is to increase the tension in that part and then suddenly release the tension.

Seitai exercises resolve partial fatigue by encouraging individuals to concentrate their attention on the specific abnormal point, while increasing the tension by using their own muscles.

Eliminating partial fatigue in the body diminishes the tired feeling throughout the entire body, leaving the body refreshed and invigorated.

HOT MOIST TOWEL METHOD

The hot moist towel method, the simple repetitive application of a hot moist towel to a troubled or painful area of the body, alleviates symptoms and effectively enhances the body's natural healing power in the following way:

(1) It immediately eases pain and discomfort.

(2) It activates the metabolism and cutaneous respiration by promoting the circulation of body fluids, such as blood and lymph.

(3) It accelerates the progress of symptoms, such as fever, by stimulating the nervous system, which controls the body's temperature.

1. Preparing a hot moist towel (Method 1)

CAUTIONARY NOTE: Take the necessary precautions to avoid scalding.
Immerse a thick face or hand towel in boiling water and wring out the excess water. Fold the towel so it is slightly larger than hand size.

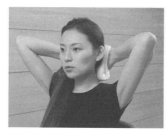

Apply a hot moist towel on the area of the body that feels painful or uncomfortable.

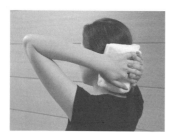

Place the hot moist towel directly on the skin.

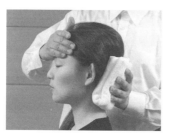

To draw a fever, the hot moist towel is applied to the back of the head.

2. Preparing a hot moist towel (Method 2)

CAUTIONARY NOTE: Use a microwave oven ONLY.

Immerse a thick face or hand towel in water, wring out the excess water and fold the towel so it is slightly larger than hand size. Heat the folded wet towel in a microwave oven until it is steaming hot. Take care when removing the towel from the microwave, as especially the underside and inside can be extremely hot.

3. How to apply a hot moist towel

The hot moist towel must be hotter than comfortably warm, but not so hot as to scald the skin. Adjust the temperature of the towel to suit individual sensitivity.

(1) Apply a hot moist towel on the area of the body that feels painful or uncomfortable. **Place the hot moist towel directly on the skin**, as the humidity of the towel promotes cutaneous respiration. It is more effective to apply a hot moist towel to the back of the head for symptoms in the eyes, ears, nose, teeth, and the head, or to draw a fever, than to apply it directly on the painful area.

(2) Reheat the towel as it cools and reapply it, repeating the process several times.

4. Mechanism of the hot moist towel method

As the hot moist towel cools quite quickly, an obvious question might be: why not use a device that maintains a constant temperature?

When a hot moist towel is applied to the body, the area covered initially tenses as a reaction to the stimulus of the heat. As the towel gradually cools, the affected area relaxes. The heating and cooling cycle achieved by repeatedly applying a hot moist towel acts as a stimulus on the body and produces the following results:

(1) It relaxes and recovers flexibility of the muscles in the affected area.

(2) It actives the metabolism by enhancing the circulation of body fluids, improving various symptoms.

(3) It enhances cutaneous respiration and perspiration of the affected area and promotes excretion of body waste.

In other words, the body reacts more to a changing stimulus, such as a hot moist towel, than a constant one, such as a heating pad. For this reason, Seitai uses the more effective hot moist towel method.

5. Drawing fever using a hot moist towel

A fever naturally rises, peaks for a short time, and then subsides to a normal temperature. When a fever is prolonged at a certain temperature, this is an indication that the body is unable to raise its temperature sufficiently high enough to peak, break, and subside.

For this reason, the individual feels discomfort, as the natural bodily reaction is restricted. In such a case, it is advisable to increase the fever further by applying the hot moist towel method. To draw a fever, the hot moist towel is applied to the back of the head.

The medulla oblongata, a part of the brain stem located at the back of the head, connects to centers that control body temperature. When a hot moist towel is held to the back of the head, the central nervous system senses the stimulus as a rise in body temperature. As a natural reaction, the body tries to radiate heat to maintain a constant body temperature. Using this method, the body's temperature first rises and then falls, leaving the body feeling refreshed and energized.

Furthermore, since functions controlling the various parts of the body are connected through the medulla oblongata, such functions are activated when a hot moist towel is applied to the back of the head. A hot moist towel is therefore effective for symptoms in the head as well as those throughout the whole body.

CYCLES IN THE BODY

Cyclical changes are fundamental to nature. Such cycles include day and night, the ebb and flow of the tides, and the changes of seasons. In harmony with these cyclical changes in nature are similar cycles of change in the human body, since human beings are part of nature. An inhalation and an exhalation is one of the shortest of such cycles, while birth and death is the longest human cycle.

A human body changes in cycles of 8 hours (6 hours in the case of serious injury or illness for adults; 4–6 hours for children), 24 hours, 3 days, 1 week, 3 weeks, 1 month, 3 months, half a year, one year, and 3 years. The 8-hour cycle has been confirmed by a recent study on the body's biological clock.

Attention should focus on the 8-hour cycle to adjust the body in daily life. When the body receives an external stimulus it begins to change in response to the stimulus. The change takes 8 hours to complete. Furthermore, the body starts to change again when another stimulus signals the start of a new cycle.

It is possible to assist the health and well-being of the body by introducing an additional stimulus at the start of a regular 8-hour cycle. Conversely, applying a second stimulus before the body's response to the first one is completed could be excessive or obstruct natural body changes. Careful attention is necessary. It is important to consider these cycles when receiving a Seitai treatment, applying the hot moist towel method, and performing Seitai exercises.

HOT BATHING METHOD

Hot bathing produces many effects, such as recovery from fatigue and adjustment of the function of the autonomic nervous system. Above all, perspiration improves, since the body perspires repeatedly during a hot bath. Activating perspiration improves metabolism, cutaneous respiration, and the body's ability to maintain constant temperature. It also strengthens the body's natural healing power and adaptability.

Kinds of hot bathing

There are five main kinds of hot bathing in Seitai:

1. Whole body bathing: soaking the entire body in hot water.

2. Foot bath: soaking the feet up to the middle of the ankles in hot water.

3. Leg bath: soaking the legs up to the knees in hot water.

4. Waist bath: soaking the lower body up to the waist in hot water.

5. Arm bath: soaking the hands and forearms up to the elbows in hot water.

The foot bath, leg bath, waist bath, and arm bath are referred to as "partial bathing." Partial bathing adds heat stimulus to only a certain area of the body. Therefore, there is a significant gap in temperature between the area being bathed and other parts of the body. Such temperature difference acts to stimulate the body and produces a greater adjusting effect on the body. As in the hot moist towel method, the gradual cooling of the bath water stimulates the natural healing power of the body. Maintaining the water temperature at a certain level therefore reduces the effect of the method.

Use the following water temperatures as a standard and adjust the water temperature in accordance with individual sensitivity, physical condition, and other individual factors. Furthermore, keep dry parts of the body warm and wipe perspiration in order to avoid body cooling.

1. Whole body bath

Seitai recommends bathing in 40–42°C water for about 5 minutes. If physically and mentally fatigued, adjust the water temperature to 39–40°C in summer (41–42°C in winter) for a longer time. When feeling only mental fatigue, take a short 2–3 minute bath in 43°C water.

2. Foot bath

Soak both feet up to the middle of the ankles in 47–48°C water for adults (45–46°C for children) for 4–6 minutes. If during that time the temperature of the water drops too much, add more hot water. The upper body should be perspiring before the end of the allocated time. If perspiration does not occur, continue bathing for another 3–4 minutes.

Both feet normally turn red after bathing. However, if one foot is not noticeably red, this would indicate that it is stiffer and less responsive to stimulation. Continue bathing that foot for an additional 2 minutes.

The foot bath is effective in improving such symptoms as a cold due to renal fatigue, abdominal hernia, coldness in the hands and feet, tonsillitis, sore throat, gynecological problems, and fatigue and pain of the legs due to physical exercise. The foot bath also eases cold symptoms before the development of a fever. Taking the foot bath in the morning normally produces the best effect.

3. Leg bath

Soak both legs up to the knees in 46–47°C water for adults (45–46°C for children). Continue bathing until the upper body starts perspiring and both legs become red. The leg bath is effective against indigestion and gastric discomfort, as well as a cold resulting from fatigue of the digestive organs. It also improves other discomfort, such as diarrhea. The leg bath is most effective if taken before going to bed. First wipe the body dry of any perspiration.

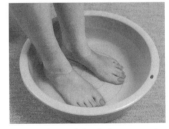

Foot bath. Soak both feet up to the middle of the ankles in 47–48°C water.

4. Waist Bath

Soak the lower half of the body up to the waist in 46–47°C water for adults (45–46°C for children) for 4–6 minutes. The waist bath is effective for unspecified discomforts below the waist arising from unidentifiable causes and difficulty recovering from a related surgical operation.

5. Arm bath

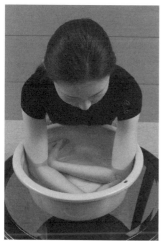

Arm bath. Soak both hands, forearms, and elbows in 46–47°C water.

Soak both hands, forearms, and elbows in 46–47°C water for adults (45–46°C for children). Continue bathing until the arms turn red. The arm bath relaxes stiffness in the ribs and pectoralis major muscles, and promotes perspiration. This bath is effective for such symptoms as bronchial disease, pneumonia, and other diseases of the respiratory system, a stiff neck after sleeping, intercostal neuralgia, and heart pain.

CAUTIONARY NOTE: The hot water temperatures indicated in this book are Seitai standards. Care must be taken to adjust water temperature in accordance with individual sensitivity.

Do NOT take a bath or shower before and/or after taking any partial Seitai bath.

Chapter 4

RELIEF FROM PAIN

HEADACHES

■ **GENERAL REMARKS**

ACUTE, SEVERE HEADACHE

Headaches can be a sign of serious problems, such as cerebral hemorrhaging, a brain tumor, among others. Careful attention to the symptoms is necessary.

CHRONIC HEADACHES

The brain's function can be seen rather like the body's version of a central processing unit (CPU) in a computer, controlling all aspects of the body. As the brain and other parts of the body are connected by a nervous system, a problem in the brain or nervous system can seriously affect the function of various organs. Conversely, problems in parts of the body can manifest as a headache.

■ **SEITAI POINT OF VIEW**

CAUSE OF HEADACHES

An examination of the body of a person suffering a headache can reveal rigidity in the neck, which obstructs blood circulation to the brain.

CAUSES OF RIGIDITY AT C1 AND C2

Rigidity at C1 and C2 is attributable to many causes, such as eyestrain, overuse of fingers and arms, lung problems, overeating, among others. These problems appear as rigidity in the related thoracic and lumbar vertebrae and are closely related to C1 and C2. Headaches experienced by women are often caused by stiffness in the pelvis.

■ SELF-TREATMENT

IMMEDIATE TREATMENT

Apply a hot moist towel 2–3 times to the upper back area of the neck.

FUNDAMENTAL TREATMENT

(a) As in any fundamental treatment, it is ideal to first determine the root cause of the headache. Even if the exact cause cannot be identified, however, the frequency and severity of headaches will be lessened by regaining the flexibility of the entire body.

(b) Improve the flexibility of the body in order to promote blood circulation. Flexibility is easily regained by practicing Seitai exercises, by receiving Seitai treatment, and most effectively when the body passes through a fever associated with a cold. Fever is a natural process of degeneration and regeneration. To suppress a fever with the use of medications obstructs this natural process and the body's ability to regain its flexibility.
Improving the entire body's blood circulation naturally enhances blood circulation to the head. At the same time, improved blood circulation accelerates metabolism and revitalizes the function of the organs, problems in which may be the source of the headache.

STRAINED BACK

■ GENERAL REMARKS

A strained back, which causes severe and sudden pain in the lower back, can occur when bending or stretching the waist.

■ SEITAI POINT OF VIEW

Though the problem can occur without warning, the cause of a strained back is long-term muscle fatigue in the area of the lower back.

The source of the strained back is mainly found in L1, L3, and L5. The muscle fatigue is caused by a variety of factors, such as habitual body movement, mental stress, overeating, fatigue of urinary organs, a problem in the sexual organs, among others. The specific cause is determined by observing the lumbar vertebrae.

Although the curvature of the lower back is determined to some extent by the environment in which the individual is born and raised, Asians, due to hereditary factors, characteristically have little curving of the lower back and the pelvis has the tendency to shift down easily. Asians therefore more commonly suffer from a strained back, as the weight of the upper body is easily transferred onto the lower back. Meanwhile, the characteristically spring-like lower back of, for example, Europeans and Africans, is relatively stronger and people from these regions less often experience lower back problems.

The spinal column in the lumbar area is comprised of five vertebrae that enable dynamic movement of the lower back. Therefore, movement of the lower back is gradually restricted as the muscles surrounding the lower back tire and stiffen. When muscle fatigue persists for a long time and exceeds a certain limit, the muscles become either extremely stiff or slack, resulting in a strained back. When this occurs, the individual is unable to move.

■ SELF-TREATMENT

Applying a hot moist towel to the aching area every eight hours stimulates the affected area in accordance with the body's hourly physical cycle of change. The hot moist towel treatment enhances such a change.

The Seitai exercise to recover a strained back relaxes the waist gradually by first working with the parts of the body the individual can move, such as the feet and legs.

■ RELAX THE SIDE ABDOMINAL MUSCLES

The waist area is supported by muscles surrounding the lumbar region and the abdomen. In the case of a strained back, the side abdominal muscles, while attempting to support the body, tend to stiffen like a plaster cast. Relaxing the side abdominal muscles will help to relax the muscles in the lumbar region and relieve the back pain.

■ PREVENTION OF RECURRENCE OF STRAINED BACK

Perform the lower back exercise daily in the morning and in the evening (see pp. 125–127).

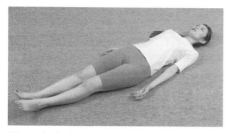

Lie on the back.

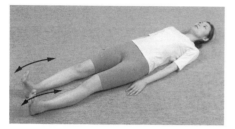

Move the feet, alternately pulling the toes toward the head and then stretching them away from the head.

EXERCISE FOR STRAINED BACK (A)

When experiencing a strained back, it is important to gradually relax the stiffened lumbar region by stimulating the moveable parts. Exercise A deals with a situation in which the sufferer experiences severe pain and inability to move. Exercise B deals with a situation in which the sufferer can achieve partial movement. Care must be taken to avoid excessive strain.

1. Lie on the back and move the feet, alternately pulling the toes toward the head and then stretching them away from the head.

2. With the legs slightly apart, alternately sway the feet outward and inward.

3. Raise the knees and draw the heels to the buttocks.

When the pain is acute, raise the knees slowly and attempt to gradually draw the heels to the buttocks.

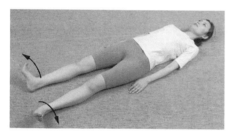
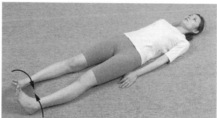

With the legs slightly apart, alternately sway the feet outward and inward.

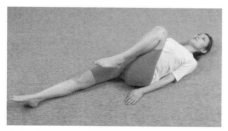
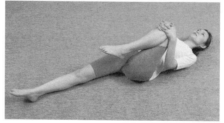

Raise the knees and draw the heels to the buttocks.

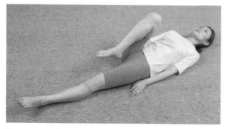
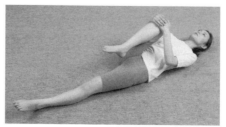

Repeating the same motion right and left alternately makes the lumbar region relaxed.

EXERCISE FOR STRAINED BACK (B)

Attempt Exercise B only after successfully completing Exercise A.

1. With the knees raised and heels drawn to the buttocks, hold the knees with both hands. Alternately bring each knee to the chest. Keep the waist on the floor.

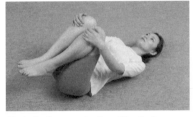

With the knees raised and heels drawn to the buttocks, hold the knees with both hands.

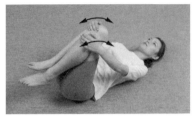

Alternately bring each knee to the chest.

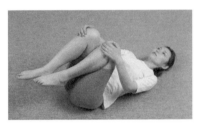

Keep the waist on the floor.

2. Extend the legs toward the ceiling and stretch the left and right Achilles tendons alternately while slowly extending the heels toward the ceiling. The calves, thighs, and backs of the knees are noticeably stretched.

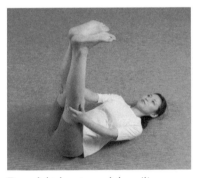

Extend the legs toward the ceiling.

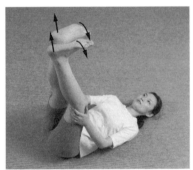

Stretch the left and right Achilles tendons alternately.

3. Spread the legs widely and lower them slowly to the floor.

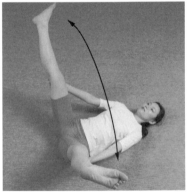
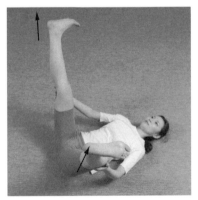
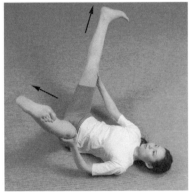

Spread the legs widely. The calves, thighs, and backs of the knees are noticeably stretched.

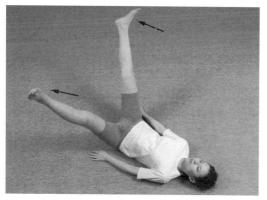 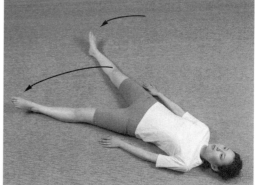

Lower the legs slowly to the floor.

SCIATICA

■ GENERAL REMARKS

Sciatica is a common type of neuralgia experienced by many people. Characteristic of sciatica is the sharp shooting pain passing through the back of the hip, thigh, and calf. As the sciatic nerve runs through the lumbar vertebrae and the back side of the leg, lumbago usually accompanies sciatic pain.

■ SEITAI POINT OF VIEW

The causes of sciatica are stiffening of the lumbar vertebrae L4 and L5, and the loss of flexibility of the pelvis.

As sciatic pain often strikes without warning, the majority of people think sciatica is an acute problem. However, acute sciatic pain occurs when the muscles supporting the lumbar vertebrae become rigid over an extended length of time and press against the sciatic nerve. As the sciatic problem deteriorates, the pain progresses down to the hip, the knee, and eventually, in the final stages, the foot.

■ SELF-TREATMENT

It is advisable to do the V-shape hip joint physical exercise, once in the morning and once in the evening, in order to loosen the ilium and the biceps femoris muscle of the thigh. After completing the exercise, apply a hot moist towel over the ilium and area of L4 and L5. If the body regains some flexibility, it is recommendable to do the L-Shape exercises and the stiff shoulder exercise to maintain flexibility (see pp. 62–64, and 130–133).

V-SHAPE HIP JOINT EXERCISE

1–2 minutes per set done once in the morning and once in the evening

1. Lie on the back. Raise the knees and draw the heels to the buttocks while raising both arms overhead. Extend and stretch the legs toward the ceiling. Rotate the legs in small circles using the hip joint as the axis of rotation.

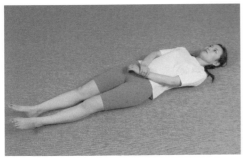

Lie on the back.

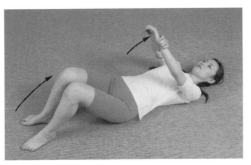

Raise the knees and draw the heels to the buttocks.

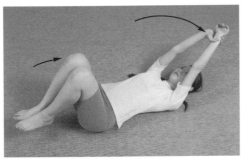

Raise both arms overhead.

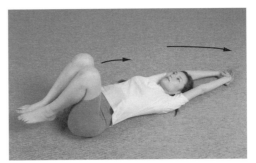

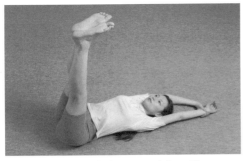

Extend and stretch the legs toward the ceiling.

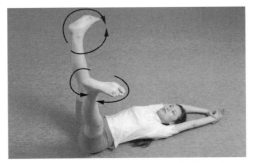

Rotate the legs in small circles using the hip joint as the axis of rotation.

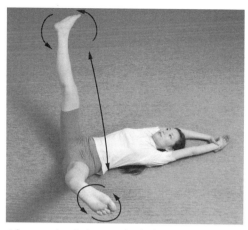

2. After rotating 3 times each clockwise and counter-clockwise, open the legs widely and rotate them in the same manner. After rotating 3 times each clockwise and counter-clockwise, hold the legs open while slowly lowering them to the floor.

3. While lowering the legs to the floor, stop the movement at the angle at which the tension is most felt in the hip joint. Rotate both legs only once clockwise and counterclockwise. Lower the legs slowly to the floor.

After rotating 3 times each clockwise and counter-clockwise, open the legs widely and rotate them in the same manner.

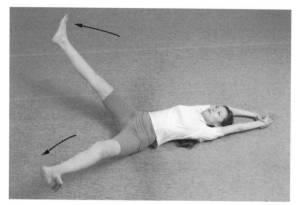
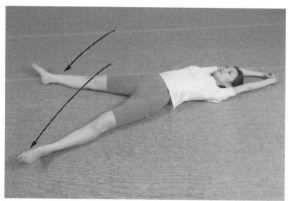

After rotating 3 times each clockwise and counter-clockwise, hold the legs open while slowly lowering them to the floor.

KNEE PAIN

■ **GENERAL REMARKS**

Considering there are many overweight people who are able to move easily and quickly without knee trouble, and slim people who have various problems in the hip joints, knees, and ankles, there would appear to be no relationship between problematic symptoms in the knees and a person's weight.

■ **SEITAI POINT OF VIEW**

Rarely is the source of trouble in a knee found in the knee itself (with the exception of a direct injury, of course). Rather, most pain in the knees originates from problems around the waist.

■ RELATIONSHIP BETWEEN THE WAIST AND THE KNEES

Lumbar vertebra L3 is closely related to the flexibility of the pelvis and twisting of the body. A knee is more easily twisted when L3 loses flexibility and thereby its ability to function properly in bodily twisting. Since the function of the knees is to bend, not twist, a knee joint becomes stiff and painful if it is twisted. This is the body's natural reaction to protect the joint from further twisting.

■ FACTORS CONTRIBUTING TO LUMBAR VERTEBRA L3 LOSING FLEXIBILITY

Aging, overeating, overworked kidneys, and excessive mental stress are some of the factors contributing to the loss of flexibility of L3.

Pain and the collection of tissue fluid around a joint are natural bodily functions to keep a joint from moving. Administering an anodyne or removing tissue fluid in the knee is simply a temporary solution to ease knee pain without determining the original cause of the problem. Such procedures could even be harmful, since the flexibility of knee joints may diminish with such repetitive treatments.

Pain in the knees can be used as a health barometer to measure problems in other areas of the body. It is important to attempt to determine the fundamental cause of knee pain when it occurs.

■ SELF-TREATMENT

Though it is necessary to determine the fundamental cause of knee pain, the discomfort can be eased to a certain extent by stretching the entire muscle along the back of the leg, including the backs of the thigh, knee, calf, and Achilles tendon, by performing a Seitai exercise specifically for knee pain (see right page). Apply a hot moist towel several times to the painful area after completing the exercise.

EXERCISE FOR KNEE PAIN

This exercise is best done on a non-carpeted surface.

1. Sit on the floor with the legs together stretched forward. Keeping the upper body straight, reach forward and place the palms and fingers of the hands over the toes. If unable to reach the toes, grasp the ankles or lower parts of the legs.

2. While pulling the toes toward the head, extend the left and right legs alternately while pushing the heels out. Keep the hips,

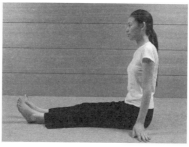

Sit on the floor with the legs together stretched forward.

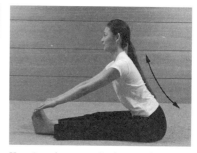

Keeping the upper body straight, reach forward and place the palms and fingers of the hands over the toes.

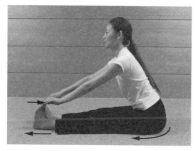

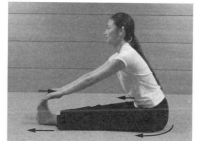

While pulling the toes toward the head, extend the left and right legs alternately while pushing the heels out.

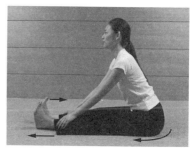

If unable to reach the toes, grasp the ankles or lower parts of the legs.

the backs of the thighs, calves, and Achilles tendons stretched. Repeat this movement slowly several times.

NOTE: This exercise is not effective unless the lumbar region is kept tensed and stretched.

HERNIATED DISK

■ **GENERAL REMARKS**

The spinal column is comprised of vertebrae separated by intervertebral disks that serve as cushions for shock. "Herniated" means "bulging" or "protruding." Hence, a herniated disk is one that has torn through its tough outer covering. If the jelly-like substance in the center of the disk protrudes far enough to press against a nerve, this can cause pain in the back as well as the legs.

The most common treatments for a herniated disk, most often the disk between L4 and L5, are stretching of the spine and prescribing pain-relieving medication.

In Seitai, the diagnosis of a herniated disk does not focus solely on the spinal column, but encompasses the entire body. As the cause of the herniated disk in the lumbar region seldom originates in the lumbar vertebrae, it is important to find the source of the symptoms and determine the fundamental solution.

For example, as in Seitai, it is generally recognized in the medical world that a relationship exists between L4 and the sexual organs, and L5 and the urinary organs. The sexual organs are easily affected by mental stress, and problems in the urinary organs tend to be caused by physical fatigue. In such cases, treatments for mental stress or physical fatigue are the fundamental solutions.

Without treating those symptoms affecting L4 and L5, the herniated disk will likely reoccur, even if focusing the treatment onto the lumbar area temporarily eases the symptoms.

■ SELF-TREATMENT

The pain of a herniated disk is eased by moving the lumbar spine while doing the physical exercise for a strained back (see pp. 43–45). Thereafter, it is advantageous to also do the L-shape exercises (see pp. 130–133).

Immediately after the symptoms start, the entire lumbar area stiffens and it becomes difficult to locate the specific affected points. Performing the aforementioned exercises relaxes the widespread stiffness and eases the ability to identify the affected points. Applying a hot moist towel to the sore area several times when the affected point is identifiable loosens the tension on those points and eases the pain.

CHRONIC LOWER BACK PAIN

■ SEITAI POINT OF VIEW

A variety of factors contribute to creating lower back pain. One such factor, for example, is the weakening of peristaltic movement in the intestines brought about by overeating.

Although it is commonly recognized that some abnormality occurring at L1, L4, and L5 is the cause of chronic lower back pain, determining the specific source of the problem without consulting a Seitai professional is difficult, since each lumbar vertebra relates to various organs in the body.

A normal spine conforms to the shape of an elongated letter "S," which provides the spinal column with spring-like power and its ability to sustain the upper half of the body.

Looking at individuals suffering from chronic lower back pain, the S-shape spine is often distorted and a greater portion of upper body weight is displaced directly onto the lumbar region, causing pain.

■ SELF-TREATMENT

Practicing the Seitai deep breathing method (see pp. 114–115) strengthens the vitality of the lower abdomen, which in turns helps to rectify the abnormality of the lumbar vertebrae and revitalize the flexibility of the lumbar region.

The side abdomen treatment is effective in relieving pain. This treatment equally benefits chronic as well as acute back pain.

In the case of chronic lower back pain, in which lumbar vertebrae L4 and L5 are compressed and press against adjacent nerves, the iliac bone exercise is an effective treatment (see pp. 123–125). Individuals experiencing problems in this area are likely to have difficulty performing this exercise owing to the accompanying pain.

After completing the exercise, apply a hot moist towel to the affected area several times. It is also good practice to apply a hot moist towel to the abdomen, since the abdominal area as well as the lumbar region often stiffens when experiencing lower back pain.

■ SIDE ABDOMEN TREATMENT

Grasp each of the side abdominal areas as though pinching them between the thumb and fingers, with thumbs on the front and fingers wrapping around the waist toward the back. While squeezing the side abdominal area, pull the hands and arms quickly away from each side without releasing the grasp, as though to pluck the side abdominal area. Repeat the movement four or five times to make one set, take a short break, and repeat again for two or three additional sets or until tension in the side abdomen is released. The squeezing and pulling action increases the strain to the affected area and the quick release relaxes the area.

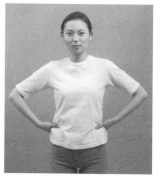

Pinch the side abdominal muscles between the thumb and fingers.

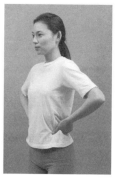

Pluck the muscles as though playing a string.

SIDE ABDOMEN TREATMENT

Pinch the side abdominal muscles between the thumb and fingers. Pluck the muscles as though playing a string, repeating 4–5 times for 1 set. Repeat for 2–3 sets with a short break between sets.

JAW JOINT DISORDER

■ **GENERAL REMARKS**

Jaw joint disorder, or temporomandibular joint disorder (TMJ), is a condition in which the individual has trouble moving the jaw or difficulty opening the mouth easily and experiences pain if an attempt is made to open it forcibly. In extreme cases, a gap of only one centimeter can be made between the upper and lower teeth.

■ **SEITAI POINT OF VIEW**

The cause of TMJ is not only problems in the bones and muscles around the jaw but also stiffness or slackness of the sternocleidomastoid muscles connecting the neck and collarbone. Furthermore, the cause of the problem in the sternocleidomastoid muscles is attributable to trouble in the lungs in most cases. In other words, the problem extends from the sternocleidomastoid muscles up to the jaw owing to the immobility of T3 and T4, which have a relationship with the lungs and the heart, respectively. In the case of TMJ, it is characteristic that the trouble in T3 and T4 reaches and affects C5 and C6 as well.

■ **SELF-TREATMENT**

As the cause of the jaw problem is often in the lungs, an attempt to only loosen the muscles around the jaw is not a fundamental solution.

To ease the symptoms of TMJ, it is recommendable to do the Seitai exercise to loosen the spinal column (see below). The basic aim of this exercise is to loosen the entire spinal column. However, the individual suffering from TMJ often experiences difficulty stretching T3 and T4. It is best to try to consciously stretch the specific part by concentrating attention to the two vertebrae.

This exercise reacts on the muscles by first tensing them and then suddenly releasing the tension. Such reaction restores the mobility of the spine and the function of the lungs recovers simultaneously.

Applying a hot moist towel on the aching part of the jaw eases the pain of TMJ.

EXERCISE TO LOOSEN THE SPINAL COLUMN

10 seconds for 1 repetition; 3–5 repetitions for one set; 2–3 sets per day.

1. Lie flat on the back, arms by the sides. Raise the outstretched arms out and over the head.

    Stretch the backbone as much as possible for 2 or 3 seconds

by extending the arms and the legs in opposing directions. Thrust the heels out as far as possible and build maximum tension in the body.

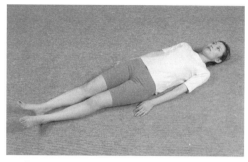

Lie flat on the back, arms by the sides.

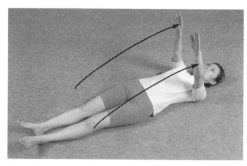

Raise the outstretched arms out and over the head.

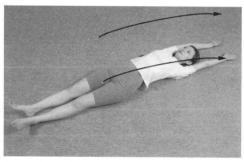

Stretch the backbone as much as possible for 2 or 3 seconds by extending the arms and the legs in opposing directions.

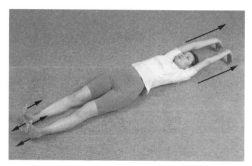

Thrust the heels out as far as possible and build maximum tension in the body.

2. Release the tension of the entire body in one sudden move.

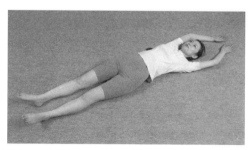

Release the tension of the entire body in one sudden move.

TOOTHACHE

■ GENERAL REMARKS

Generally, the source of a toothache is recognized to be a buildup of bacteria.

■ SEITAI POINT OF VIEW

The source of a toothache, even in the absence of tooth decay, is found in the ilium. There is a correlation between the position of the ilium and the health of teeth.

A common symptom seen in individuals suffering from toothache is a descending and stiff ilium. This tendency is apparent especially in individuals fitted with dentures.

The downward shift of the ilium, caused mainly by physical fatigue, disrupts the balance of the nervous system and the skeletal structure, manifesting as toothache. For the same reason, swelling of the gums is experienced when one is very tired.

Tooth decay occurs when blood circulation in the head is diminished by sagging of the occipital area resulting from a downward shift of the ribs and ilium. This reduces the strength and vitality of the teeth and gums.

■ SELF-TREATMENT

To ease an acute toothache, apply a hot moist towel to the upper neck at C1 and C2. Since this area is vital in terms of promoting blood circulation to the head, it is more effective to apply the towel to this region than directly to the area around the aching tooth.

Though the Seitai physical exercise for the ilium (see pp. 123–125) is designed to ease the movement of the lumbar region, it also effectively alleviates a toothache by increasing flexibility in the lumbar region and related lung area at the same time.

HEMORRHOIDS

■ GENERAL REMARKS

Hemorrhoids, swollen veins in the area of the anus, are caused by excessive tension in the anal area leading to congested blood circulation in the area. The main symptoms of hemorrhoids are swelling around the anus and protrusion of the swelling to the inside and outside of the anus. The affected area is often inflamed, painful, and itchy, and rectal bleeding occurs in some cases.

■ **SEITAI POINT OF VIEW**

Hemorrhoids are caused by a weakening in the function of the heart. While there would appear to be little relationship between the heart and hemorrhoids, as the two regions are physically distant, the decline in the function of the heart's ability to pump blood throughout the body results in weakened blood circulation in such extremity as the anus. Hence, blood congestion causes the various symptoms of hemorrhoids to emerge.

Characteristic of individuals suffering hemorrhoids is that T4, which relates to the function of the heart, is dull. If the condition deteriorates, then T3, which is related to the respiratory organs, also loses flexibility. From this Seitai viewpoint, abnormalities of the heart and the respiratory organs are the origin of hemorrhoids.

■ **SELF-TREATMENT**

To ease hemorrhoid pain associated with a bowel movement, apply a hot moist towel directly to the anus. Although common advice for treatment of hemorrhoids is to bath the lower half of the body, the repetitive heating and cooling stimulus of the hot moist towel method more effectively enhances blood circulation than does keeping the area at a constant temperature for a certain time.

In order to recover the function of the heart, it is recommendable to do the Seitai physical exercise that stimulates T3 and T4.

To determine the fundamental solution, it is necessary to find the source of abnormality of T3 and T4. In some cases, this is attributable to poor perspiration.

The ilium exercise or C-shape exercise (see pp. 123–125 and pp. 138–139) which promote the function of the heart, are effective in most cases.

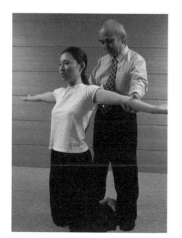

EXERCISE FOR T3 AND T4

Recovering the flexibility of T3 and T4, which are related to the lungs and heart respectively, enhances the function of these organs.

1. Stand on bent knees and raise both arms forward and up over the head and gradually lower laterally to a horizontal position, palms facing up. Expand the chest, which moves the shoulder blades closer together.

2. Extend the left and right arms alternatively, keeping the move-

ment slight and slow so as to avoid moving other parts of the body. Focus on increasing the tension in the area of T3 and T4.

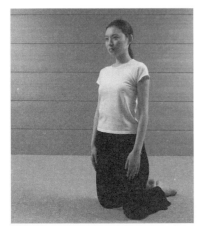

Stand on bent knees.

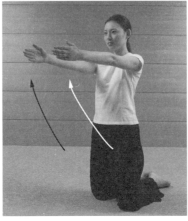

Raise both arms forward and up over the head and gradually lower laterally to a horizontal position.

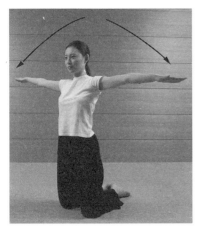

Keep the palms facing up.

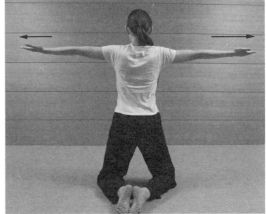

Expand the chest, which moves the shoulder blades closer together.

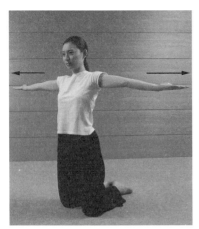

Extend the left and right arms alternately.

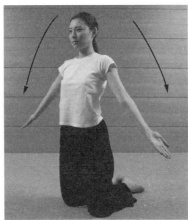

Lower the arms slowly.

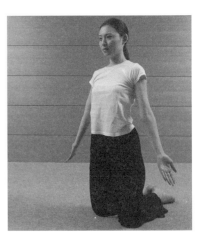

GOUT

Gout, a form of acute arthritis, is inflammation caused by excessive levels of uric acid in the blood and the resulting accumulation of urate crystals in the affected joints. In the past, gout was associated with the wealthy, who frequently ate rich food and drank to excess. Nowadays, the most common sufferers of gout are males between 40 and 50 years old. Women are less likely to suffer gout before menopause, owing to the difference in their hormonal composition.

The main symptoms of gout are sudden severe pain, swelling, and tenderness most frequently occurring at the base of the big toe. The pain is so acute that it is called gout spasm.

■ SEITAI POINT OF VIEW

The excessive nutrition from overeating (related to T7, T8, and T9), and a decline in the function of the heart (T4) and the kidneys (T10) are regarded as the causes of gout.

Uric acid accumulates easily because of the deterioration of blood circulation attributable to a functional decline of the heart. The kidneys are also unable to efficiently filter body waste and the level of uric acid, which normally passes through the kidneys and into the urine, accumulates in the joints in the form of urate crystals.

■ SELF-TREATMENT

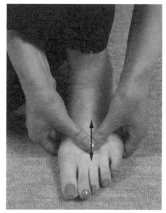

Grasp the foot with both hands, fingers around the sides and onto the sole, and wedge the thumbs in the space between the bones.

It is recommendable to do the technique to expand the gap between the bones in the forepart of the feet in order to excrete urate crystals accumulated at the joints. This is done by grasping the foot with both hands, fingers around the sides and onto the sole, and separating the bones by wedging the thumbs in the space between the bones. Apply DOU-KI with the thumbs on stiff or contracted areas. It is more effective to expand the gap from the forepart of the foot to the base of the foot.

After completing the technique, taking a footbath helps to promote blood circulation and enhances the excretion of uric acid.

The circulation of blood throughout the body is a closed system connected by blood vessels. Therefore, if blood circulation at the extremities is weak, the body's entire blood circulation is affected. Conversely, promoting blood circulation at the extremities improves the blood circulation of the whole body.

RHEUMATISM

■ GENERAL REMARKS

In the first stage of rheumatism, joints in the hands and fingers stiffen in most cases and the individual experiences difficulty in grasping objects firmly. As the condition deteriorates, pain is felt even when the joints are motionless. However, a greater concern than the pain of rheumatism is the gradual stiffening and deformation of the joints, which restricts joint movement, and the subsequent spread of the disease throughout the entire body.

■ SEITAI POINT OF VIEW

The cause of rheumatism is the accumulation of waste elements in the joints as a result of the decline in the function of the heart, related to T4, and thereafter the liver, spleen, and kidneys, related to T7 through to T10. The liver, kidney, and spleen play crucial roles in the detoxification of the body, which is significantly affected by blood flow from the heart. If the flow of blood is irregular, the normal function of these three organs is likely to be impeded, as blood needs to pass steadily through these organs for proper detoxification.

■ SELF-TREATMENT

The combined exercise (see p. 127–129) is recommendable to promote the excretion of waste elements. Moreover, the lymphatic exercise (see pp. 118–123) and C-shape exercise (see pp. 138–139) relax the body and normalize the heart's function. If the symptoms are acute, the exercise to loosen the spinal column is recommended (see pp. 52–53).

Partial bathing can help to ease the pain and promote blood circulation. First, a foot bath (water at 116–118°F [47–48°C] for adults) taken twice a day, after waking and before going to bed, promotes circulation throughout the entire body.

Soak the individual aching parts of the body in hot water (114–116°F [46–47°C] for adults). If an elbow aches, take an arm bath. The effect of the arm bath is strong, sometimes producing a feeling that the body is dull and heavy. This expected reaction, however, indicates that the body is relaxed.

CAUTIONARY NOTE: Those who have extremely weak lungs should avoid taking an arm bath too often and for a long period of time.

STOMACH CRAMPS

■ GENERAL REMARKS

Stomach cramps is a broad term used to describe spasmodic pain occurring in and around the stomach. The cause of stomach cramps is difficult to pinpoint, since the related pain can arise from a simple inflammation of the stomach or from a variety of more serious ailments, such as gallstones, acute pancreatitis, stomach ulcers, a duodenal ulcer, a pyloric ulcer, etc.

■ SEITAI POINT OF VIEW

The main cause of stomach cramps is overeating and excessive mental stress. More so than any other part of the body, the stomach is easily affected by mental factors and the influence of excess mental stress. Overeating causes the stomach to first expand beyond its normal limit before contracting to its original size. This process creates stomach cramps.

■ SELF-TREATMENT

In most cases of stomach cramps, the upper gastric area aches first and the pain thereafter moves to the pit of the stomach, which tightens and cools. Applying a hot moist towel on this area is effective treatment.

Performing DOU-KI (see p. 60) on the pit of the stomach effectively enhances KI, improves blood circulation, and eases stomach pain.

The rib tightening method promotes the function of the stomach and at the same time relaxes the stiff intercostals, eases breathing, and alleviates the pain of the cramps.

RIB TIGHTENING METHOD

NOTE: This method requires the assistance of a second individual.

■ EFFECTS: ALLEVIATES STOMACH CRAMPS

The sufferer lies on his or her back. The assistant extends the sufferer's right arm away from the body and takes a kneeling position parallel to the sufferer's right side at the ribs. The assistant raises the sufferer's left knee and places the left foot flat on the floor. The assistant gently brings his or her own right knee against the sufferer's ribs along the right side of the body and gently cups the ribs along the left side of the body with both hands. The assistant carefully and lightly squeezes the ribs toward the central axis of the body.

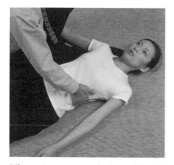

The assistant extends the sufferer's right arm away from the body and takes a kneeling position.

DOU-KI

1. GASHO GYOU-KI

Practicing GASHO (palms facing one another) GYOU-KI enhances the flow of KI in the palms of the hands.

1. Squat down as in the illustration or sit on the edge of a chair with the back fully erect. Position the hands' palms facing at a distance of about 10cm. Close the eyes lightly, relax, and take deep breaths, as if inhaling and exhaling from the finger tips.

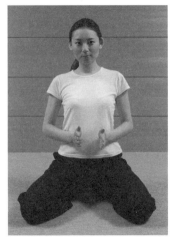 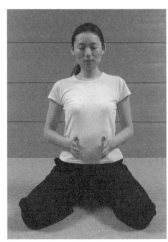

Squat down and position the hands' palms facing at a distance of about 10cm.

Close the eyes lightly, relax, and take deep breaths.

2. Continue such breathing for a few minutes, noting that sensations may arise between the palms and fingers, such as warming, cooling, pulsations, the feeling of magnetic attraction and repulsion, etc.

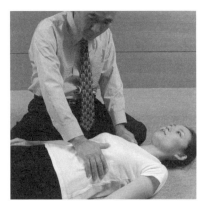

Apply the hand with enhanced KI flow on a painful or uncomfortable area of the recipient's body. Concentrate your attention on that point. Imagine inhaling and exhaling from the palm of the hand.

2. DOU-KI

Apply the hand with enhanced KI flow on a painful or uncomfortable area of the recipient's body. Concentrate your attention on that point, and imagine inhaling and exhaling from the palm of the hand. DOU-KI can also be done by oneself.

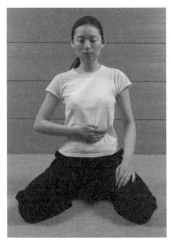

DOU-KI can also be done by oneself.

Chapter 5

EASING DISCOMFORT

STIFF SHOULDERS

■ **GENERAL REMARKS**

Stiff shoulders occur when the muscles from the neck to the shoulders tighten, resulting in a heavy, dull feeling in the area.

The muscles around the shoulders continuously sustain the weight of the arms, unless the body is in a horizontal position. When the muscles supporting the arms lose strength or when excessive force is applied to the shoulders because of skeletal distortion, the shoulder blades first lose flexibility and then the muscles around the shoulders stiffen, resulting in obstructed blood circulation and the occurrence of pain in the area.

■ **SEITAI POINT OF VIEW**

The source of shoulder trouble is not in the shoulder, but is caused by overeating, overuse of the arms, hands and fingers, eyestrain, etc., which first creates an abnormality in the lumbar region. The discomfort of stiff shoulders is attributable to the abnormality of the lumbar vertebrae extending through the back and chest to the shoulders.

In other words, when the pelvis shifts downward and distorts, the scapulae shift laterally outward and away from the spine, and the back stiffens. Owing to this distortion, the weight of the arms pulls down on and compresses the chest and shoulder area. If the lumbar is sufficiently flexible, such distortion does not occur.

As the fundamental cause of stiff shoulders does not originate in the shoulders, the most effective treatment is a physical exercise that stimulates the entire spinal column.

The stiff shoulder exercise relaxes the shoulders by first increasing the tension in the shoulders and the spinal column, and then quickly releasing the tension. This exercise also helps to effectively raise the pelvis and correct distorted posture.

When the cause of stiff shoulders is attributable to the digestive organs, it is advisable to use the SANRI technique (see p. 64), which acts on the vital point of the digestive organs.

To ease acute shoulder pain immediately, apply the hot moist towel method to the aching area.

EXERCISE FOR STIFF SHOULDERS

1. In a standing position, keep the legs straight and lean the upper body slightly forward. Arch the lumbar region and then straighten the upper body. This will bring tension into the lower back and the top edge of the ilium.

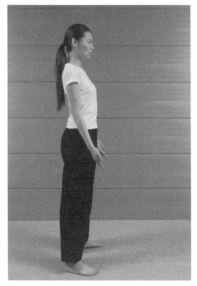

Stand naturally.

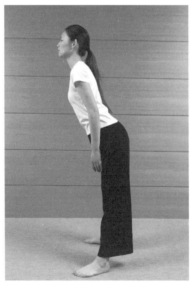

In a standing position, keep the legs straight and lean the upper body slightly forward.

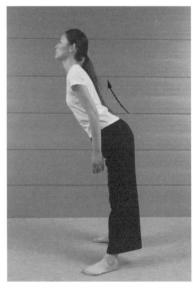

Arch the lumbar region and then straighten the upper body.

2. While raising both arms slowly forward, palms facing up, bend slightly forward from the waist. Do not spread the arms wider

than shoulder width, keep the palms horizontal, and hold the tension in the spine and lower back.

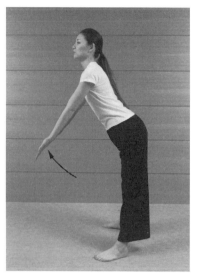

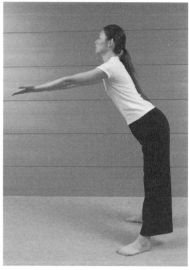

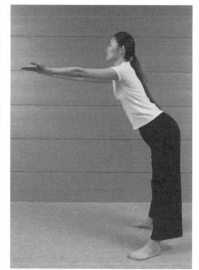

While raising both arms slowly forward, palms facing up, bend slightly forward from the waist.

Do not spread the arms wider than shoulder width, keep the palms horizontal, and hold the tension in the spine and lower back.

3. Maximum strain is felt in the spinal column and shoulders at the angle at which the arms cannot be raised further. Alternately extend each arm 2–3 times. Lower the arms slowly while returning to an upright position.

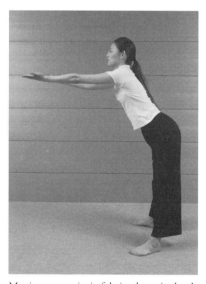

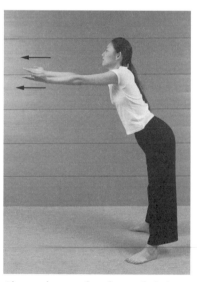

Maximum strain is felt in the spinal column and shoulders at the angle at which the arms cannot be raised further.

Alternately extend each arm 2–3 times. Lower the arms slowly while returning to an upright position.

Be sure to avoid the following incorrect postures:

1. The lumbar is not arched.
2. The arms are spread too wide.
3. The palms are not facing up.

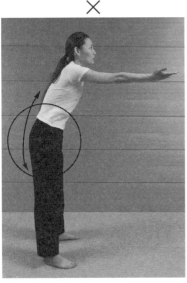

The lumbar is not arched.

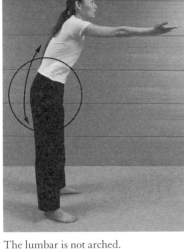

Correct posture.

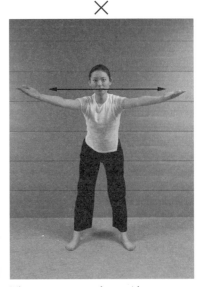

The arms are spread too wide.

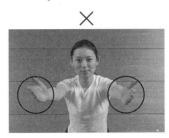

The palms are not facing up.

SANRI

Stimulating SANRI, a vital point in the muscles of the forearms that stimulates the digestive organs, is effective treatment for stiff shoulders caused by problems in the digestive organs due to overeating. When overeating, a node appears in SANRI which, when stimulated, produces a sharp, resonating pain that helps to relax shoulder stiffness.

SANRI is a stiff point on the muscle near the elbow on a line between the elbow and the thumb. Pinch SANRI between the thumb and fingers and then pluck the muscles, repeating 3–4 times.

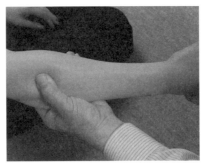

SANRI is a stiff point on the muscle near the elbow on a line between the elbow and the thumb.

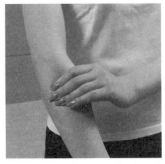

Pinch SANRI between the thumb and fingers and then pluck the muscles, repeating 3–4 times.

SHOULDER PAIN CAUSED BY AGING

■ GENERAL REMARKS

Shoulder pain experienced by middle-aged people in Japan is called "shoulder pain of the 40s" or "shoulder pain of the 50s," owing to its frequent appearance in people of these age groups. This form of shoulder pain is characterized by the inability to move the shoulder freely and pain created when the shoulder is moved.

■ SEITAI POINT OF VIEW

Although various symptoms in the shoulders are generally confused as shoulder pain caused by aging, the symptoms of such shoulder pain from the Seitai perspective are:

(1) Limited ability to extend the arm behind the body.

(2) Constant pain that does not get progressively worse.

(3) The patient recovers after a period of three months despite undergoing no treatment.

Western medical science tends to diagnose all forms of stiff and painful shoulders as one and the same problem. From the Seitai perspective, the two are distinctly different.

The pelvis drops as the body ages, and this can cause a distortion in the body's balance. Seitai believes that the body's attempt to regain balance creates the shoulder pain.

Stiff shoulders are expressed along the spinal column at vertebrae (1) C7 and T1, which are related to the arms, (2) T3 and T4, which are related to the lungs and heart, or (3) T6–8, which are related to the digestive organs.

■ SELF-TREATMENT

It is important to warm the body by taking a bath to ease the pain. For optimum results, soak the body in 104–109°F (40–43°C) water for 10 minutes.

The breastbone physical exercise (see pp. 115–118) and stiff shoulder exercise (see pp. 62–64) alleviate stiffness around the shoulder blades and pelvis. Though it might at first be difficult to perform these exercises owing to the severity of the shoulder pain, the pain will diminish through perseverance.

If the intensity of the pain prevents attempting the exercises, first apply a hot moist towel to the painful area.

SHOULDER JOINT PAIN

■ **GENERAL REMARKS**

The symptom of shoulder joint pain is sharp pain in and around the shoulder joint. Seitai categorizes it separately from the dull discomfort experienced with stiff shoulders and shoulder pain in older individuals.

Characteristically, only the shoulder joint aches and the pain intensifies day by day. The pain occurs even while sleeping and it can at times be so sharp as to awaken the individual.

The cause of the pain is the accumulation and solidification of calcium around the shoulder joints, which irritates the surrounding muscles and creates more pain. If no attempt is made to move the shoulder joint, more calcium accumulates and the pain intensifies.

■ **SEITAI POINT OF VIEW**

The accumulation of calcium around the shoulder joints is caused by the deterioration of blood circulation, which is related to the heart. Excessive amounts of elements, like calcium, do not accumulate when the heart functions normally.

■ **SELF-TREATMENT**

Shoulder joint pain often occurs suddenly and can be intolerable. If doing a Seitai physical exercise to ease the pain is difficult, first apply the hot moist towel method to the affected area. Note, however, that the basic Seitai principle is to apply a hot moist towel *after* performing an exercise, since the stimulus of an exercise would disperse the concentrated effect produced by the hot moist towel method.

The purpose of the recommended shoulder exercise is to relax the stiff muscles in the affected shoulder joint that have wound excessively tight around the joint as a natural defensive reaction against the painful stimulus of the calcium.

Sufferers may at first be reluctant to move the aching shoulders, but once the stiffened muscles around joints become flexible and loosen from the bone, the shoulder joint is able to recover to its normal condition.

SHOULDER JOINT EXERCISE

Various muscles converge at the shoulder joint. Pain or discomfort is felt when the arm is positioned at angles that tense the related stiff-

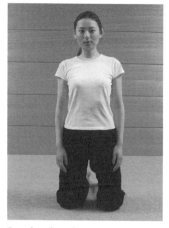

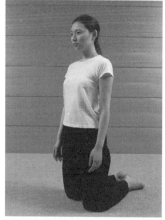

Stand on bent knees.

ened muscles. This exercise recovers the movement of the shoulder joint by relaxing the stiffened muscles.

1. Stand on bent knees. Make a loose fist with the thumb extended. Raise and bend the arm forward, bringing the thumb to rest on the shoulder. Keeping the thumb on the shoulder, raise the elbow straight up as high as possible.

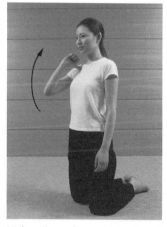

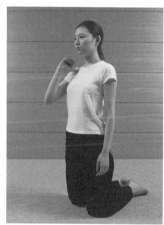

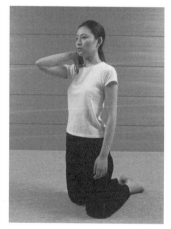

Make a loose fist with the thumb extended.

Raise and bend the arm forward, bringing the thumb to rest on the shoulder.

Keeping the thumb on the shoulder, raise the elbow straight up as high as possible.

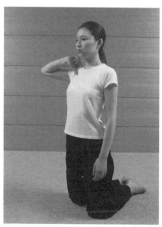

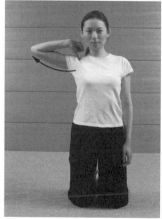

With the elbow at maximum height, swing slowly the bent arm out toward the side of the body.

2. With the elbow at maximum height, swing slowly the bent arm out toward the side of the body.

3. Extend the arm and stretch it upward at the angle that creates the most tension in the shoulder joint. At the same time, open the fist finger by finger, starting from the forefinger.

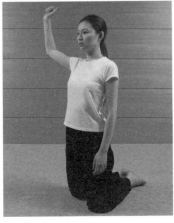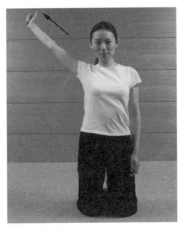

Extend the arm and stretch it upward at the angle that creates the most tension in the shoulder joint.

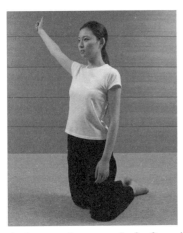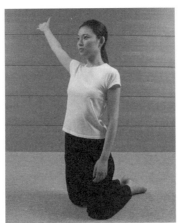

At the same time, open the fist finger by finger, starting from the forefinger.

4. Rotate the arm clockwise and counter-clockwise using the shoulder as the axis of rotation. Find the position at which the force concentrates most strongly in the shoulder joint.

5. At the position of greatest concentration of force, extend the arm as far as possible to stretch the stiffened shoulder. At maximum tension, release suddenly.

6. Stretch the arm out lightly at the same angle again and direct it downward while extending it behind the body. If an obstruction is felt at a certain position during the movement, repeat Step 5.

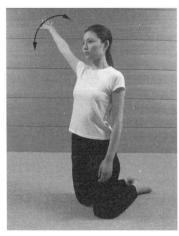

Rotate the arm clockwise and counter-clockwise using the shoulder as the axis of rotation.

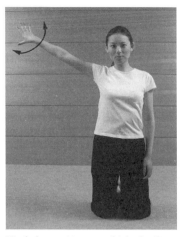

Find the position at which the force concentrates most strongly in the shoulder joint.

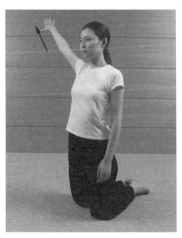

At the position of greatest concentration of force, extend the arm as far as possible to stretch the stiffened shoulder.

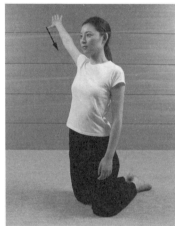

At maximum tension, release suddenly.

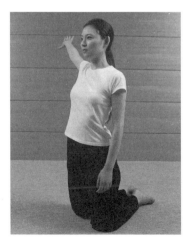

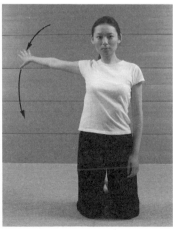

Stretch the arm out lightly at the same angle again and direct it downward while extending it behind the body. If an obstruction is felt at a certain position during the movement, repeat step 5.

OTHER SHOULDER JOINT PAIN

■ SEITAI POINT OF VIEW

Various types of shoulder pain exist other than those caused by aging or the accumulation of calcium.

Shoulder joint pain is most commonly caused by lung compression due to excessive load. The compressed lung causes the head of the humerus (top of the upper arm bone) to shift from its normal position, causing pain.

The cause of pain is determined by identifying the painful area:

(1) Acromion (a bone extending from the scapula around the shoulder joint at the rear to form a roof over the humerus): overuse of the arms.

(2) Head of the humerus (front side): abnormality in the lungs and arms.

■ SELF-TREATMENT

Overuse of arms: exercise for stiff shoulders (see pp. 62–64). Abnormalities in the lungs and arms: breastbone exercise (see pp. 115–118).

It is recommendable also to do the exercise for shoulder joint (see pp. 66–69) in addition to the above exercises.

EYESTRAIN

■ GENERAL REMARKS

Eyestrain, characterized by eye tiredness or pain around the eyes, is caused by overuse of the eyes. The source of this symptom could simply be eye fatigue, or the sign of a disorder in another part of the body.

■ SEITAI POINT OF VIEW

In Seitai, the brain and the eyes are thought of as one unit, with the eyes representing the part of the brain that is exposed. The condition of the brain is reflected in the eyes so that the response of the pupils is used as a standard to determine brain death. Eye symptoms can therefore be interpreted as some form of brain disorder.

The brain functions continuously and easily tires, at which point the skull shifts down and presses against the optic nerves, manifesting as eye trouble.

One method of self-treatment is to stimulate the medulla oblongata, which from the Seitai perspective is related to the optic nerves, by rotating the eyes. Repeat the movement and observe near and distant objects. This exercise can improve the activity of both the eyes and optic nerves as well as the function of the brain. Also effective is to firmly press the temples and cheekbones in toward the center of the face and to pull the earlobes. At times of acute pain, apply a hot moist towel over the closed eyes and temples. This method can help to improve eyesight and reduce eyestrain.

APPLYING DOU-KI ON THE CLOSED EYES IS ALSO EFFECTIVE.

The most important thing is to rest the eyes. The eyes are not meant to endure stress such as that created by looking at a PC monitor for an extended period of time. The ability of the eyes improves by alternately using them in moderation and resting them when they are not used.

DRY EYE

■ GENERAL REMARKS

People are seldom conscious of tears unless they flow from the eyes. However, the surface of the eye is kept moist and dust-free by the fluid secreted from the tear glands, which also provides nutrition to the conjunctiva and cornea, the outermost layers of the eyeball.

Dry eye is a generic name for problems caused by the lack of secretion of tears. The main symptoms of dry eye are as follows:

(1) Eye irritation and eye pain.

(2) Eye fatigue.

(3) Difficulty opening the eyes.

(4) Increased blinking.

(5) Excessive eye mucus.

(6) Bloodshot eyes.

■ SEITAI POINT OF VIEW

There are two causes of dry eye:

(1) The body's ability to expel waste becomes deficient.

(2) The muscle controlling the tear glands becomes dull.

In other words, the cause of dry eye is a decline in the body's ability to secrete sufficient tears, and problems in the muscle controlling the quantity of tears. In addition, attention should be given to the shifting down of the occipital area, which is related to the eyes.

■ SELF-TREATMENT

To recover normal tear secretion, it is vital to regain and revitalize physical strength to efficiently expel unnecessary body waste.

As secretion is closely related to perspiration, the body needs to perspire easily to recover proper secretion. The now prevalent use of air conditioning in the hot summer months has resulted in people perspiring far less in recent years. As a result, the body's natural function to sweat when in a hot environment is not responding efficiently.

The purpose of sweating is to excrete body waste and to adjust the body's temperature. Therefore, the body's inability to sweat efficiently exerts an additional burden on other organs responsible for excretion, which weakens the excretion ability of the entire body.

Sweating efficiently during hot weather increases the mobility of T5, which is related to perspiration. This produces a positive effect on T4, related to the heart, and likewise promotes the function of the muscles controlling the tear glands.

Placing a hot moist towel and performing DOU-KI on the closed eyes can help to temporarily ease the pain and discomfort of dry eye.

INSOMNIA

■ GENERAL REMARKS

The following are generally recognized as symptoms of insomnia:

(1) Inability to sleep well, even at night.

(2) Waking up too early.

(3) Sleeping for a sufficient length of time, but feeling fatigued or a sense of discomfort, as though not having slept, since the sleep is too shallow.

■ SEITAI POINT OF VIEW

Sleep is recognized as necessary to recover energy. In other words, sleep is an important form of "nutrition" absorbed by the body, similar to eating food. While sleep is important, it should be noted that the purpose of human life is *to be actively doing something* rather than sleeping and eating. Indeed, sleeping and eating supply the body with the nourishment it needs to be active. As an individual develops an appetite for food when hungry, the body needs the "nutrition" of sleep when it is moderately tired.

When one wakes earlier than normal, it is evidently because the individual has had a sufficient amount of sleep. Careful attention should be taken when the ability to sleep is inhibited by excessive body tension caused by extreme fatigue of a part of the body or of the entire body. In such cases, it is advisable to make efforts to improve one's lifestyle or the entire constitution of the body according to Seitai principles and practice.

Sleep gives the body rest by relaxing the entire body. Taking sleeping medication to get to sleep dulls bodily functions and does not achieve a natural state of rest.

A relationship exists between the depth of sleep and depth of breathing. The pectoralis major muscles of someone unable to relieve fatigue, despite getting sufficient sleep, are often tense. This makes breathing shallow and inhibits sound sleep. Therefore, the body does not fully recover from physical fatigue and the brain also is unable to recover from mental fatigue.

■ SELF-TREATMENT

The parts of the body related to breathing, such as the pectoralis major muscles, the thorax, and the intercostals, must be relaxed.

The exercise to ease the tension of the pectoralis major muscles, the exercise to lift the ribcage (see below), and performing DOU-KI to the upper chest area are all effective for producing a sound sleep. Applying a hot moist towel on the upper chest around the sternoclavicular joint before going to bed also helps to improve the quality of sleep.

EXERCISE FOR THE PECTORALIS MAJOR MUSCLES

This exercise recovers the flexibility of the pectoralis major muscles, which stretch across the upper chest on both the left and right sides, using the weight of the arm and the force of the outstretched arm. Stretching each muscle is more difficult than usual if this exercise is attempted when tired.

1. Stand on bent knees. If releasing tension in the right pectoralis major muscle, slowly rotate the right arm in a clockwise move-

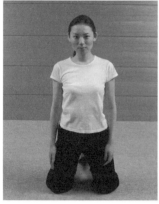
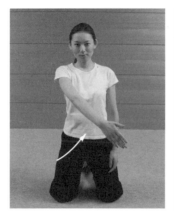

Stand on bent knees.   Rotate the arm across the front of the body up over the head.

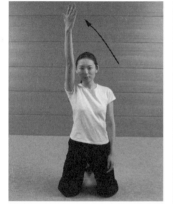
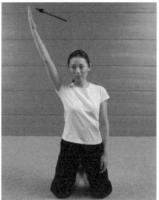
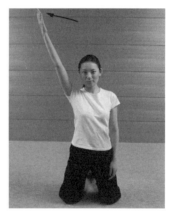

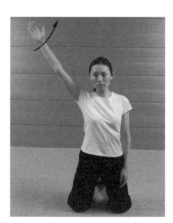
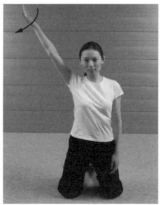

Gently rotate the arm clockwise and counter-clockwise, focusing on angling the arm to bring maximum tension along the arm and the chest.

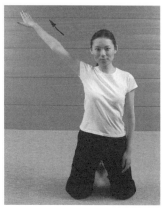

Stretch the fingers, thumb, and arm fully at the angle that brings maximum tension along the arm and the chest. Hold the tension in the muscle for a short time and release sharply.

ment across the front of the body, up over the head, and down toward the right and slightly behind the body. Keep the hand open and especially stretch and extend the base of the palm and the thumb while gently rotating the arm clockwise and counterclockwise, focusing on angling the arm to bring maximum tension along the arm and the chest.

2. Stretch the fingers, thumb, and arm fully. If the arm is properly stretched, the force and weight of the arm will also stretch the pectoralis major muscle. Hold the tension in the muscle for a short time and release sharply.

3. Stretch the arm again and lower it while rotating it behind the body.

4. Repeat the same steps with the left arm for the left pectoralis major muscle.

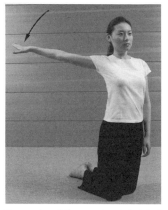

Lower it while rotating it behind the body.

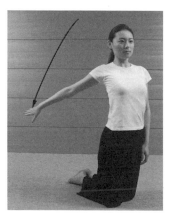
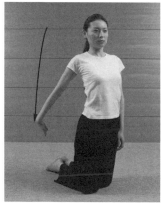
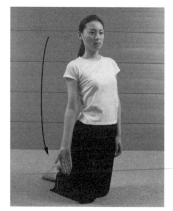

EXERCISE TO LIFT THE RIBS

This exercise relaxes the muscles around the chest by using the weight of the arm. If the muscles around the chest relax, the fallen ribs rise, breathing deepens, and sleep improves.

1. Lie on the floor on the left side of the body. Extend the arm against the floor out and over the head and in line with the body, using the arm as a headrest. Slightly bend the right knee and place the right arm along the right side of the body. Rotate the hand counter-clockwise until the thumb points behind the body.

2. Rotate the right arm counter-clockwise, focusing on stretching the muscles around the chest. Relaxing the arm and fully utilizing the weight of the arm more easily stretches the muscles. Adjust the angle of the right leg in order to maintain body balance.

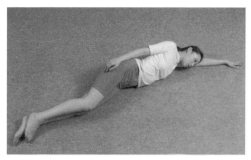

Lie on the floor on the left side of the body. Extend the arm against the floor out and over the head. Slightly bend the right knee and place the right arm along the right side of the body.

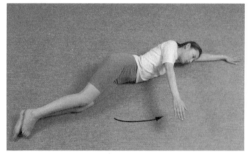

Rotate the hand counter-clockwise until the thumb points behind the body.

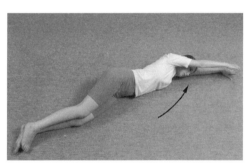

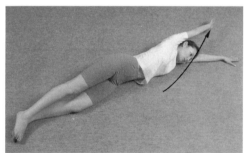

3. Stretch the arm in the direction of the arrow (see photo at right) at the point of maximum tension.

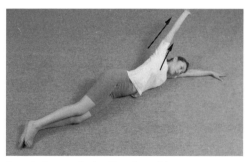

Stretch the arm in the direction of the arrow.

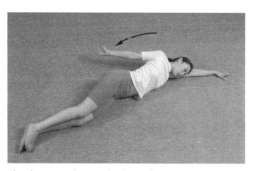

Slowly rotate the arm backward.

4. Slowly rotate the arm downward and backward.

5. Repeat the steps lying on the right side of the body to relax the left chest muscles.

STIFF NECK AFTER SLEEPING

■ **GENERAL REMARKS**

Generally, a stiff neck is thought to be caused by an excessive strain applied to the neck as a result of, for example, sleeping on a pillow that is too soft.

■ **SEITAI POINT OF VIEW**

Seitai theory believes that the cause of a stiff neck, rather than a pillow or something external to the body, is found within the body itself. A body in good condition relaxes while sleeping. However, if a problem exists somewhere in the body, that part of the body alone remains tense during sleep, and the disparity of tension in the body manifests as a stiff neck upon waking.

Moreover, overeating can also be the cause of a stiff neck. Overeating exerts an excessive burden on the digestive organs, which stiffens thoracic vertebrae T6 (related to the stomach) and T7 (digestive organs). Stiffness in T6 and T7 has an effect on the neck (cervical vertebrae) and the discomfort in the neck affects the appetite. Hence, an individual with a stiff neck due to overeating generally loses appetite. From the Seitai perspective, a stiff neck is the natural function of the body to provide rest for the digestive organs.

The neck is a vital part of the body, since it supports the head and connects it and the brain to the rest of the body. Therefore, excessive massaging or manipulation of the neck is not recommended, since the neck muscles, although they initially soften after a massage, afterward become even more stiff and dull. In a like manner, the skin on the palms of the hands and the soles of the feet becomes tough when constantly stimulated.

■ **SELF-TREATMENT**

It is effective to do the combined exercise (anti-overeating and activating lymph; see pp. 127–129) to dissipate the burden on the digestive organs and revitalize their functions. The twist and stretch exercise (see below) is also effective for easing the symptoms.

Applying the hot moist towel method to the aching part of the neck after doing the exercises also helps to relieve the discomfort.

TWIST AND STRETCH EXERCISE

1. Lie on the back.

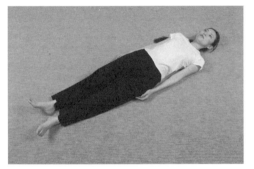

Lie on the back.

2. Raise and extend both arms overhead.

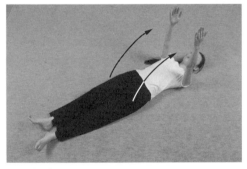

Raise both arms.

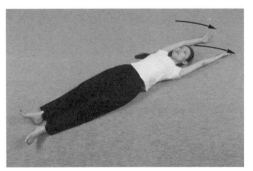

Extend both arms overhead.

3. Stretch the left half of the body using the left arm and the left leg. Pull the toes toward the head and extend the heel. Before stretching the arm, rotate it clockwise and counter-clockwise, extending and loosening the base of the palm, and hold it at the position of maximum tension. Stretch the leg and arm out as

much as possible, slightly adjusting their angles so as to increase tension in the left side of the body.

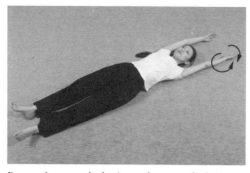
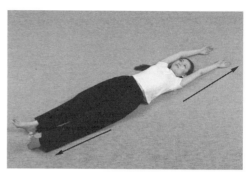

Rotate the arm clockwise and couter-clockwise to find an angle making maximum tension to the body.

Stretch the leg and arm out as much as possible.

4. Release the tension suddenly. Repeat the same steps on the right side of the body.

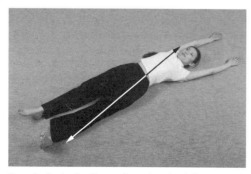

Release the tension suddenly.

5. When the body cannot be stretched sufficiently using the above method, stretch the body diagonally using the left arm with the right leg and the right arm with the left leg.

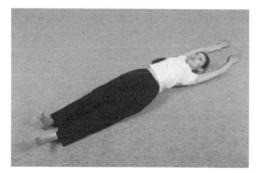
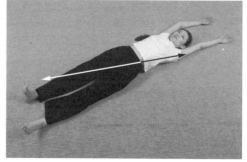

Stretch the body diagonally using the left arm with the right leg.

Stretch the body diagonally using the right arm with the left leg.

DIARRHEA

■ **GENERAL REMARKS**

Diarrhea is characterized by frequent, loose bowel movements, but the symptoms can differ from one person to another. Under healthy circumstances, a stool that is soft for one individual may seem quite normal for another. Therefore, careful attention to the symptoms is needed. In general, diarrhea is more frequent excretion than usual of soft or watery excrement.

The most common causes of diarrhea are infections from bacteria, viruses, or parasites, or the effect of mental stress on hypersensitive intestines.

■ **SEITAI POINT OF VIEW**

Seitai rarely regards diarrhea as a sickness. Rather, diarrhea is viewed as a normal bodily function to rid the body of unnecessary materials. In other words, diarrhea occurs when the body needs to excrete unnecessary or potentially harmful substances. Therefore, diarrhea should normally not be suppressed and instead be left to run its course until the excretion is complete. One exception, however, is diarrhea caused by a blow to the head, which can be serious and needs careful attention.

■ **SELF-TREATMENT**

When diarrhea is severe to the extent that it places excessive stress on the body, an attempt should be made to ameliorate the symptom. In such severe cases, the body becomes hypersensitive to a variety of internal and external stimuli and over-reacts. The exercise to loosen the spinal column (see pp. 52–53) helps to ease the symptoms of diarrhea by relaxing nervous tension in the body.

When diarrhea is severe and accompanied by a stomachache, apply a hot moist towel on the aching area of the abdomen, which also helps to ease the cramping discomfort felt in the area. A hot moist towel applied to the abdomen is especially effective for diarrhea caused by mental stress. While determining the exact cause of diarrhea might require professional assistance, it can to some extent be determined by carefully reflecting on one's circumstances in daily life.

Soaking the legs up to the knees in 115–117°F (46–47°C) water (cooler for children) is an effective treatment for diarrhea associated with a cold. Add more hot water frequently as the water cools, but keep the water level below the knees. The variance in the air and water temperatures stimulates the body and causes blood vessels in the legs to expand and contract repeatedly, which more effectively promotes circulation than if the water were maintained at a constant temperature.

ATHLETE'S FOOT

GENERAL REMARKS

Athlete's foot is a condition that affects the spaces between the toes. The early signs and symptoms of athlete's foot include itching, stinging, and burning between the toes, and later blistering, cracking and peeling of the skin, especially between the toes and on the soles of the feet. The condition can spread to the toenails and other parts of the body. Though typically more common among men, women are becoming increasingly afflicted with this problem.

■ **SEITAI POINT OF VIEW**

Athlete's foot is caused by the deterioration of lymph circulation. According to western medical science, athlete's foot is caused by infectious microscopic fungi, the most common known as *trichophyton rubrum*. However, if lymph circulation is normal and the immune system functions properly, the body does not become susceptible to such fungal infection.

When the heart experiences difficulty, lymph circulation also deteriorates. The symptoms of poor lymph circulation first appear at the body's extremities. The feet are an area of the body where internal body waste easily accumulates and becomes the source of trouble.

■ **SELF-TREATMENT**

To improve the symptoms of athlete's foot, it is important to dry the body fluid in the affected area and improve the circulation of body fluids. An easy method of drying the affected area, especially the spaces between the toes, is to use a hair drier. Avoid applying a hot moist towel on the affected area.

Expanding the gap between the bone (see p. 57) in the forepart of the feet improves the circulation of body fluid in the feet. Practicing the C-shape physical exercise (see pp. 138–139) improves the function of the heart, relaxes the entire body and, as a result, promotes the circulation of body fluids.

As treatment for athlete's foot, professional Seitai practitioners manipulate the pubic bone, which is a vital point for any skin trouble from the Seitai perspective.

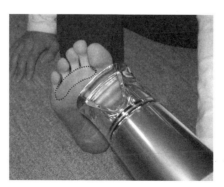

Use a hair drier to dry the affected area between the toes.

MENTAL STRESS

■ **GENERAL REMARKS**

Stress is ubiquitous in modern society and many people suffer from excessive mental stress. Psychiatric or psychological counseling is a common approach to treating this problem.

■ **SEITAI POINT OF VIEW**

The breathing of an individual suffering mental stress is extremely shallow and restricted to the upper chest. At times, the person's shoulders move up on inhaling and down on exhaling.

Meanwhile, the center of gravity of a physically and mentally healthy individual remains below the navel, the point Seitai calls the lower tanden. The inhalation seemingly extends to the base of the abdomen, and the individual has a dignified and calm disposition.

Tolerance to mental stress differs from one individual to another. If two people are subjected to the same degree of stress, one might remain calm, while the other might become extremely restless and irritated. In Seitai, mental stress and physical flexibility are considered to be closely related. A physically tense individual suffers various symptoms, and is unable to deal effectively with external stress. Relaxing the mind is difficult as long as the body is tense, even though one resorts to various medicinal and non-medicinal treatments, as such treatments generally address only the mental faculty.

■ **SELF-TREATMENT**

Relaxing the body is the most effective way to relax the mind. The thumbs of the hand and the large toes of the feet are vital points related to the brain. Excessive stress causes these extremities to stiffen. Pulling and rotating the thumbs and large toes helps to relax and loosen them. This method is effective as a first aid treatment to relieve sudden mental stress in daily life. Applying a hot moist towel to the tensed part of the chest or pit of the stomach is also an effective temporary treatment.

The physical exercise to loosen the spinal column (see pp. 52–53) is an effective fundamental treatment. In this exercise, the entire body is first stretched to its maximum using the limbs and, thereafter, the tension is suddenly released. This method of inducing maximum tension followed by sudden release of tension relaxes the entire body.

The deep breathing method (see pp. 114–115) may be difficult to perform, but it is effective for the individual with shallow breathing.

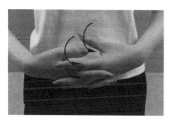

Interlock the fingers and rotate the thumb alternately.

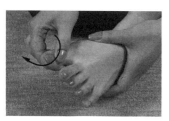

Rotate the big toes.

ROTATING THE THUMBS AND BIG TOES

Interlocking the fingers and rotating the thumbs alternately helps to soothe the mental condition. Rotating the big toes eases tension in not only the big toes and the feet but also the entire body.

SWELLING OF THE FEET

■ **GENERAL REMARKS**

Swelling, or edema, normally occurs in the body's extremities, such as the hands and, more commonly, the feet. In the feet, the symptoms include a heavy, dull feeling, and the sensation that the shoes are small and fit tightly.

■ **SEITAI POINT OF VIEW**

Swelling is linked to blood circulation problems caused by weak blood and body fluid circulation, and the accumulation of waste elements. The primary causes of the symptoms are deterioration of the function of the heart and/or the weakening of the function of the kidneys and liver, which filter and detoxify the blood and eliminate waste elements.

Although the heart pumps blood, carrying oxygen and nutrients through arteries throughout the body, the pumping pressure of the heart does not extend to all the veins in the extremities. Instead, muscle contraction acts to compress the veins and to help move the blood, containing carbon dioxide and body waste, back to the heart.

Swelling often occurs when the body's muscles (and organs) are tired and lose flexibility due to standing or working for prolonged periods of time. The leg muscles less effectively move the blood up the body and the heart is unable to maintain a normal level of blood circulation.

■ **SELF-TREATMENT**

Relaxing the joints, which are the gateway of bodily fluid circulation, promotes smooth blood circulation in the lower half of the body.

Firstly, relax the ankle joints by doing the physical exercise to relax the ankles (see next page). A footbath also helps to ease swelling. Secondly, it is recommendable to do the L-shape exercise (see pp. 130–133) to relax the ilium in order to promote blood circulation in the entire lower half of the body. The lower half of the body contains 2/3 of the body's muscles. Therefore, moderate daily movement of the lower half of the body by walking, for example, improves the circulation of the entire body.

To improve the function of the heart itself, relax T3 and T4 and the chest by doing the breastbone exercise (see pp. 115–118), the exercise for T3 and T4 (see pp. 55–56), and/or the C-shape exercise (see pp. 138–139).

EXERCISE TO RELAX THE ANKLES

30 seconds for 1 repetition; 2–3 repetitions per set; 2–3 sets per day

1. Sit on the floor with the legs extended forward. Grasp the ankles with the hands. Move the toes toward and away from the head.

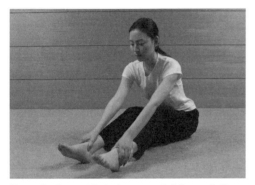

Sit on the floor with the legs extended forward. Grasp the ankles with the hands. Move the toes toward and away from the head.

2. It is also effective to grasp the ankle with the hand and rotate it.

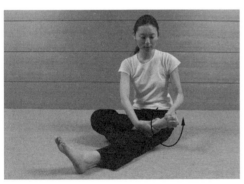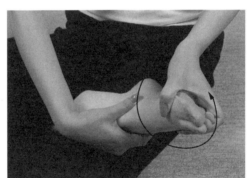

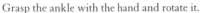

Grasp the ankle with the hand and rotate it.

Chapter 6

IMPROVE YOUR CONDITION

COMMON COLD

■ GENERAL REMARKS

The symptoms of a cold include fever, chills, joint pain, headaches, runny nose, coughing, sneezing, sore throat, nausea, and diarrhea. Although viruses like influenza cause some colds, the root cause of most colds remains unknown.

A common treatment for cold symptoms is prescribed medicine, such as an antipyretic (an agent that prevents, removes, or allays a fever) or a lozenge. Recently, however, the danger of suppressing the symptoms of such illnesses as influenza encephalitis (inflammation of the brain) using medicines, such as an antipyretic, is becoming more widely recognized. The medical world is increasingly becoming aware of the importance of allowing the common cold to be cured through a natural process without medication. From the Seitai point of view, this trend is most appropriate.

■ SEITAI POINT OF VIEW

In Seitai, a cold is not regarded as an illness. Rather, a cold is viewed as a natural bodily function that adjusts a disorder and recovers the body to its normal healthy condition.

If an individual is unable to rid the body completely of fatigue experienced in daily life, fatigue gradually accumulates in the body. The area of the body affected by fatigue varies according to the individual's lifestyle, habitual use of the body, and other individual characteristics.

A cold is an outward manifestation of the symptoms of accumulated body fatigue. By undergoing the process of a cold, the accumulated fatigue is eliminated and the entire body is refreshed.

While it might seem incongruous, a healthy body is one that catches a cold easily. A cold symptom can be extremely subtle and, in some cases, a cold can pass with just a few sneezes. An individual with such a sensitive body rarely suffers from a serious illness, since physical problems arise and disappear virtually unnoticed.

On the contrary, a body that seldom catches a cold is regarded as unhealthy, since such a condition would indicate that the body's sensitivity to dormant problems is dull. When a person with such a body catches a cold, the symptoms are serious and the recovery time is lengthy. In extreme cases, a critical or potentially life-threatening illness could suddenly develop.

Since a cold is a process of adjustment, it is vital that the process be natural, that no attempt be made to stop the symptoms, and that all the problems be eliminated from the body.

The ideal time to catch a cold is during the change of seasons, when the body adapts its condition to deal with the change in temperature, humidity and dryness in accordance with the season's change. By means of a cold, the sensitive body attempts to eliminate problems accumulated in the previous season as preparation for the coming season.

■ SELF-TREATMENT

When symptoms of the respiratory system appear, an elbow bath offers effective relief. Problems of the respiratory system affect the arms, which stiffen as a result of the burden placed on the lungs. An arm bath relaxes the arms and elbows, which eases breathing and relieves coughing. A leg bath helps to relieve a stomachache associated with a cold and a footbath is recommended to ease a sore throat.

Expanding the chest eases cold symptoms that affect the respiratory system, such as coughing. For this purpose, the breastbone exercise (see pp. 115–118) is recommended. The lymphatic exercise (see pp. 118–123) increases metabolism and accelerates the process of a cold. The L-shape exercise (see pp. 130–133) relieves lower back pain. The illiac bone exercise (see pp. 123–125) relieves lower back pain and also recovers the functions of the lungs and heart

A hot moist towel is normally applied to the area of the body where discomfort is felt. However, for symptoms in the head, the towel can be applied to the back of the upper neck.

When a fever stagnates near 100°F (38°C) and is prolonged, it is recommendable to raise the fever by applying the hot moist towel method to the back of the upper neck. This temporarily increases the body's temperature to around 102–104°F (39–40°C), after which the temperature decreases to normal.

After experiencing a high fever, the body's temperature will decrease to below normal temperature. **It is essential to rest until the body's temperature recovers to its normal level.**

HAY FEVER (POLLINOSIS)

■ **GENERAL COMMENTS**

Generally, hay fever is regarded as an allergic response to the pollen of various plants and trees that vary by country and area. Though hay fever caused by cedar pollen flourishes in Japan with the onset of spring, individuals recently have been suffering allergic reactions throughout the year, excluding winter.

■ **SEITAI POINT OF VIEW**

The cause of hay fever is not the pollen, which appears with the onset of spring, but the inability of the body to properly adjust to the change of season.

Normally, the body loses flexibility as temperatures decrease in the fall and winter and it regains flexibility with the arrival of warmer spring weather. If a part of the body is unable to regain flexibility in springtime, symptoms of the body's attempts to relax the stiffened parts appear as, for example, a runny nose and sneezing.

Individuals who suffer hay fever symptoms all year round (excluding winter) demonstrate stiffness in the entire body. Such bodies are unable to adjust to even slight, yet alone normal, changes of the seasons, and the various types of allergic symptoms arise in order to promote the adjustment.

■ **SELF-TREATMENT**

The exercise to loosen the spinal column (see p. 52–53) is effective for loosening a stiff body. For a hay fever sufferer, this exercise is initially difficult.

It is also recommendable to do the lymphatic exercise (see pp. 118–123) or breastbone exercise (see pp. 115–118) to relax the ribs and the exercise for thoracic vertebrae T3 and T4 (see pp. 55–56).

To relieve eye itchiness and watering, apply the hot moist towel method directly on the closed eyes. And to calm a runny nose and sneezes, apply the hot moist towel method to the back of the head.

Taking an arm bath is also recommended when the symptoms are especially severe.

ENERGY LOSS

■ **GENERAL REMARKS**

Energy is the source of activity and power to live. When energy declines, sexual desire decreases first.

Decline of sexual desire normally occurs in middle-aged and older individuals as a natural process of aging. However, so-called "sexless" young couples have been increasing in number recently. Their ability to function sexually is normal, but they do not have a sense of sexual desire.

■ **SEITAI POINT OF VIEW**

The pace of life in modern society is producing excessive mental stress. From the Seitai point of view, the cause of decreased sexual desire is the decline in function of the respiratory system due to excessive mental stress, which often occurs when a person is discouraged or disappointed. During such a time, the posture of the individual often droops forward, which places a burden on the lungs that impedes their ability to function normally. This condition affects T3 and T4, which are related to the lungs and the heart, respectively. T3 and T4 are related to L4, L5, and S2, which are related to the sexual organs and the cause of the decline of sexual desire.

■ **SELF-TREATMENT**

If energy decline becomes apparent, it is recommendable to do the exercise to loosen the spinal column (see pp. 52–53) in the morning and at night. The brain is connected to the body's internal organs and muscles through the nervous system. Relaxing the spinal column smoothes the transmission of brain signals and enhances the function of the internal organs and muscles, including the secretion of sex hormones.

Continuing this exercise relaxes the body that has contracted as a result of mental stress. As the body becomes able to more easily handle mental stress, the adverse effect on the respiratory system will also dissipate.

The illiac bone exercise (see pp. 123–125) is designed to relax the

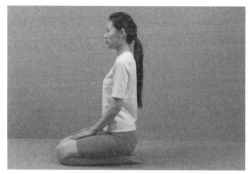

Sit in a kneeling position.

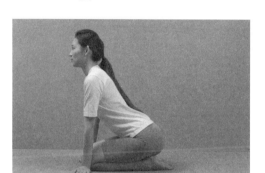

Use the arms and hands for support.

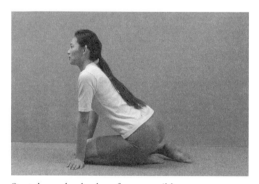

Stretch one leg back as far as possible.

pelvis, which contains the internal sexual organs and relates to the lungs. This exercise also helps to prevent energy loss.

The hip joint physical exercise effectively counters energy decline attributed to aging. This exercise makes the hip joint flexible, where indications of aging appear earlier than in other parts of the body, by promoting lymph circulation in the lower half of the body. The exercise also helps to prevent energy loss as well as hypertrophy (excessive growth) of the prostate gland.

HIP JOINT EXERCISE

The symptoms of aging most often first appear in the hip joints. Symptoms of the lumbar region and the urinary organs tend to appear more frequently when a hip joint stiffens. Keeping the hip joints flexible helps to prevent aging.

1. Sit in a kneeling position. Using the arms and hands for support, stretch one leg back as far as possible. Slide the bent knee of the opposite leg forward to ease the stretching.

2. Put weight on the hip joint of the stretched leg and stretch the hip joint. Adjust the angle and/or positioning of the feet and toes until maximum tension is brought into the hip joint.

3. Keep the posture for 10–20 seconds.

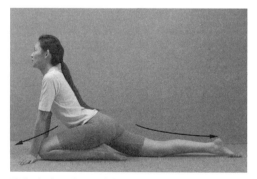

Slide the bent knee of the opposite leg forward to ease the stretching.

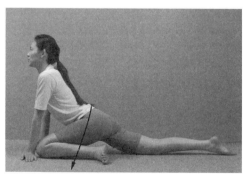

Put weight on the hip joint of the stretched leg and stretch the hip joint.

POOR COMPLEXION

■ GENERAL REMARKS

The following are recognized medically as the causes of poor complexion:

1) ANEMIA.

Anemia is a condition in which the blood is deficient in red blood cells, in hemoglobin, or in total volume.

2) BLEEDING.

Chronic bleeding attributed to hemorrhoids, ulcers of the stomach and duodenum, stomach cancer, uterine cancer, etc.

3) HEART / PULMONARY DISEASE.

Owing to an insufficient supply of oxygen in red blood cells, the blood vessels appear black and blue, and the complexion looks pale.

4) KIDNEY DISEASE.

The complexion looks pale owing to a swelling of the face.

5) LEUKEMIA.

A condition similar to anemia, leukemia is characterized by an abnormal increase in white blood cells in the tissues of the body.

■ SEITAI POINT OF VIEW

Since there are people with a pale complexion who are healthy, it is necessary to determine the individual's natural skin complexion under normal, healthy conditions. Generally, the cause of a poor complexion is poor blood circulation of the entire body owing to the stiffening of T3 and T4, which are related to the lungs and the heart, respectively.

The complexion of an individual with low blood pressure or anemia tends to be pale, while that of an individual with high blood pressure tends to be red. In Seitai, more attention is given to the gloss of the face than to its color. Lack of skin luster may be an indication of a problem with the internal organs. In addition, mental factors should also be considered when assessing skin complexion.

■ SELF-TREATMENT

It is recommendable to relax body stiffness and improve blood circulation by doing the exercise to loosen the spinal column (see pp. 52–53). Furthermore, it is advisable to normalize distortion in the body, especially rib stiffness, by doing the lymphatic exercise (see pp. 118–123) and the C-shape exercise (see pp. 138–139). These exercises will help to improve the function of the heart, which is encased in the ribs, as well as the complexion of the skin.

An individual with a poor complexion generally has a stiff body and will initially have difficulty doing these exercises. It is also advisable to do the deep breathing method (see pp. 114–115) together with these exercises.

Applying a hot moist towel to the extremities, such as the hands and feet, will improve circulation in those areas and help to promote circulation throughout the entire body.

HEART PALPITATIONS (ARRHYTHMIA)

■ **GENERAL REMARKS**

People are not usually conscious of their own heartbeat, since heartbeats are generally regular and steady. Therefore, arrhythmia, commonly known as heart palpitations, which are characterized by faster-than-normal, slower-than-normal, or irregular heartbeats, is immediately noticed. Other than fluctuation in the rhythm of the heartbeat, heart palpitations are often noticed when the individual becomes hypersensitive to the heartbeat due to mental problems or has a pathological condition known as tachycardia (relatively rapid heartbeat).

Rapid heartbeat felt after exercising or when emotionally excited is natural in most cases. From the medical perspective, the following are the main examples of disease accompanied by abnormal heartbeat:

1) BASEDOW'S DISEASE.

Associated with hyperthyroidism, heart palpitations may occur at times when the body requires a large quantity of oxygen owing to accelerated metabolism as a result of increased levels of thyroxin, a thyroid hormone.

2) ANEMIA.

Due to the lack of oxygen-carrying red blood cells, the heart beats more rapidly to send oxygen throughout the body.

3) HEART DISEASE.

Problems in the muscles or valves of the heart may upset the regular flow of blood.

■ **SEITAI POINT OF VIEW**

In those cases where heart palpitations are acute or occur often, it is necessary to seek the assistance of a doctor or Seitai professional to determine the source of the symptoms.

When there is no problem in the function of the heart itself, the following other factors can obstruct the function of the heart in most cases:

(1) The stomach is distended due to overeating. As a result, the chest is constricted.

(2) Exertion on the heart attributable to an abnormality in the respiratory system (T3 & T4; L4). Excessive mental stress is sometimes the source of such trouble in the respiratory organs.

Heart palpitations require special and careful attention, as they can at times be the sign of a life-threatening problem.

■ SELF-TREATMENT

Relaxing the entire body by doing the C-shape exercise (see pp. 138–139) improves metabolism. As a result, the function of the heart is enhanced and the palpitations are alleviated.

If the exercises are too difficult to attempt or their effect does not soon become apparent, it is recommendable to consult a specialist in order to determine the source of the problem.

Applying the hot moist towel method on the center of the chest relaxes the area constricted by mental stress or overeating and recovers the function of the heart.

HIGH BLOOD PRESSURE

■ GENERAL REMARKS

Blood pressure is a measure of the amount of blood pumped by the heart and the amount of resistance to blood flow in the arteries. High blood pressure develops when blood pressure rises to an abnormally high level due to problems in the heart and/or arteries.

Maximum blood pressure is measured when the heart contracts to pump blood and minimum blood pressure is measured when the heart is momentarily at rest and the arteries are expanded by the flow of blood from the heart.

An individual is diagnosed as having high or low blood pressure based on World Health Organization (WHO) guidelines.

In Seitai, an individual's numerical blood pressure reading is not compared against the WHO average. As tall people, for example, tend to have high blood pressure, Seitai takes individual factors into consideration, such as the person's height and weight, when considering what a normal blood pressure reading would be for each individual.

High blood pressure occurs when the thorax contracts, as a result of mental stress or overeating, and obstructs the function of the heart, or when thickening and hardening of arterial walls (arteriosclerosis) impedes blood circulation.

A characteristic physical feature of an individual with high blood pressure is the protrusion of T8. If the individual were to back up slowly to a wall, he or she would first feel T8 press up against the wall.

■ SELF-TREATMENT

The most common cause of high blood pressure is overeating. Overeating causes the extended stomach to exert pressure on the heart and blood circulation is abnormally accelerated in order to digest the large quantity of ingested food. In such cases, it is necessary to curb overeating, including taking snacks between meals.

It is recommendable to do the combined exercise (lymph exercise and the exercise for overeating, pp. 127–129), which promotes the function of the digestive organs and relaxes the thorax. If the individual has difficulty doing this exercise, it is recommendable to first attempt the lymphatic exercise (pp. 118–123) done lying on the back.

INDIGESTION

■ SEITAI POINT OF VIEW

Indigestion is attributed to overeating and an extremely tired stomach. Ingesting more food before the previously ingested food is completely digested puts a strain on the capacity of the stomach and intestines, causing indigestion. Furthermore, the digestive organs, such as the stomach and intestines, are easily affected by mental stress. The symptoms of indigestion often appear when the individual has a work-related concern or a family problem.

Daily life can be stressful and an individual may not always be able to eliminate the cause of stress by oneself. Therefore, Seitai assumes that people cannot escape the mental stress of daily life and instead aims at creating a flexible body capable of receiving and dealing with stress properly without producing adverse effects.

■ SELF-TREATMENT

The most effective treatment to relieve indigestion is to rest the stomach by reducing the quantity of food eaten for approximately one week.

It is recommendable to do the combined exercise (see pp. 127–129) to recover the function of the over-exerted digestive system. An overeater generally has a stiff body, and reclining the upper body backward will likely be difficult at first. It is necessary to be aware of the body's limitations and avoid forceful straining.

The hot moist towel method is effective relief for a stomachache caused by indigestion. Applying the hot moist towel on the pit of the stomach eases the pain of the stomachache and promotes digestion at the same time.

Refer to the section on mental stress (see pp. 82–83) for information concerning building resistance to stress.

PSEUDO MYOPIA—FALSE NEARSIGHTEDNESS

■ GENERAL REMARKS

Individuals who have difficulty seeing things in the distance, but not in close range, have a condition known as myopia, or nearsightedness. Pseudo myopia, or temporary nearsightedness, is recognized as eyestrain resulting from focusing on nearby objects for an extended period of time.

■ SEITAI POINT OF VIEW

The main source of eye trouble is distortion of the ilium, such as dropping of the ilium and left-right imbalance. The ilium is related to the occipital region of the back of the head, which also shifts down. Furthermore, such movement in the occipital region exerts pressure on C1, C2, and C3, supporting the optic nerves, thereby affecting eyesight. The eyes provide a glimpse of the mental state of the individual. Therefore, pseudo myopia, in addition to eye trouble, may indicate mental fatigue.

■ SELF-TREATMENT

Pseudo myopia improves comparatively easily with proper early treatment, since it is a temporary symptom. It is recommendable to first do the iliac bone exercise (see pp. 123–125) and the L-shape exercise (see pp. 130–133) to rectify the condition of the ilium. If the effects of

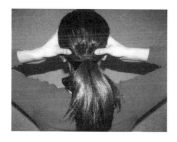

these two physical exercises do not appear distinctively, it is advisable to lift the occipital region using both hand (see photo at left).

Moreover, it is necessary in daily life to attempt to maintain a proper posture by remaining conscious of the arch of the lumbar vertebrae. A proper posture raises the ilium, which produces a beneficial effect on eyesight.

Applying the hot moist towel method on the closed eyes stimulates the flexibility of the eyeballs and improves the symptoms of pseudo myopia.

CHRONIC FATIGUE

■ GENERAL REMARKS

Chronic fatigue, characterized by the feeling of being perpetually tired, is a result of the inability of the individual to get rid of accumulated body fatigue. The source of chronic fatigue varies from physical to mental factors. The following diseases are recognized as the causes of chronic fatigue:

1) DIABETES.
Glucose in the bloodstream is not adequately absorbed and the blood sugar level rises.

2) LIVER TROUBLE.
When hepatic function weakens, metabolic change and detoxification stagnate.

3) BERIBERI.
Owing to the lack of thiamine (vitamin B1), absorption of glucose into the blood is weakened.

4) NEUROTIC ILLNESSES.
When an individual suffers from neurosis or a nervous breakdown, the will to motivate oneself is often lost.

■ SEITAI POINT OF VIEW

When it is clear that the individual has one of the above problems, treatment of the causes of the problems is necessary.

Although everyone experiences fatigue, chronic fatigue occurs through the individual's inability to eliminate fatigue accumulated in the body. The causes of the symptoms are an extreme lack of physical strength and endurance. The body of an individual with chronic fatigue is characteristically very stiff. In other words, in order to remove the fatigue, it is necessary to relax the muscles stiffened by the fatigue. The person suffering chronic fatigue, however, is in a weak condition to attempt to relax the muscles.

Fatigue induces sleep, which in turn eliminates fatigue. But when the entire body is excessively tired, the ability to sleep can be impaired.

Currently, partial fatigue, characterized by extreme tiredness of only a part of the body (mental or physical), is not uncommon. In such a condition, even sleep is unable to alleviate such partial fatigue.

■ SELF-TREATMENT

The shimo-tanden (lower tanden), located in the lower part of the abdomen, reveals one's physical strength. When the individual is healthy, the shimo-tanden is full of power and the whole body, especially the lumbar area and pelvis, is flexible and mobile. As a result, breathing is very deep.

The Seitai breathing training called shinsoku-ho (see pp. 114–115) is an effective technique for strengthening the shimo-tanden. Practicing this breathing method increases physical strength and recovers flexibility of the lumbar area. The individual builds resistance to fatigue and is able to recover from fatigue more rapidly.

The breathing of individuals who tire easily is shallow, and such breathing places a burden on the body. By practicing shinsoku-ho, the body becomes accustomed to deep breathing, and the individual increases resistance to mental stress. This indicates that the body has the ability to accept and manage external stimuli by itself.

CONSTIPATION

■ GENERAL REMARKS

The symptoms of constipation vary by individual. Even if bowel movements are frequent, the individual is constipated if the bowel movement takes an extremely long time or the colon and rectum do not feel completely void. Conversely, an individual is not constipated if bowel movements are less frequent and yet the individual feels no discomfort and encounters no difficulty in daily life.

■ SEITAI POINT OF VIEW

The cause of constipation is weakening of peristalsis of the intestines as well as the stomach. In a normal condition, the intestines and stom-

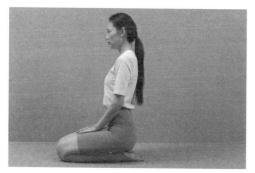
Squat on the floor.

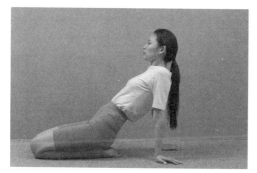
Recline back over the lower legs and rest the back on the floor.

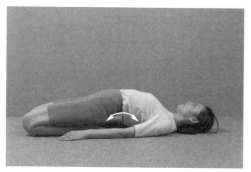
Keep the legs and feet from shifting to the outer sides of the hips.

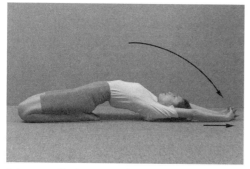
It is more effective to raise both hands over the head.

ach start peristalsis (related to T6, T10, and T11) when the body needs nourishment, and this movement evacuates the waste (related to L2). However, an excessive burden placed on the stomach and intestines over an extended period of time adversely affects their functions and weakens peristalsis. This causes constipation.

■ SELF-TREATMENT

First, reduce food intake in order to recover gastrointestinal function. Although the feeling of hunger may be difficult to endure, it stimulates the stomach and intestines and activates their functions. Gastrointestinal function is enhanced when small quantities of food are ingested after a sufficient period of hunger. Owing to the activated peristalsis, feces that might have been lodged in the intestines for a long time, and which can cause various problems in the body, are excreted.

The Seitai exercise for overeating helps to determine the degree of overeating in an individual. At the same time, the exercise also effectively promotes the function of the digestive organs.

If the symptoms of constipation are acute, it is recommendable to do the exercise for constipation. In this exercise, the movement of the foot is used to stimulate the colon, located in the lower left abdomen, and the rectum, and to promote the function of the intestines.

When a stomachache develops, applying the hot moist towel method on the lower abdomen eases the pain and promotes evacuation.

EXERCISE FOR OVEREATING

1. Squatting on the floor, recline back over the lower legs and rest the back on the floor. Keep the legs and feet from shifting to the outer sides of the hips.

2. It is not possible to attempt this posture if the digestive organs are overworked due to overeating. The lumbar region of the back arching too far from the floor, or the knees lifting from the floor and spreading apart indicate possible overeating.

3. It is more effective to raise both hands over the head.

EXERCISE TO RELIEVE CONSTIPATION

Stimulate the function of the descending colon in the lower left abdomen and the rectum using the movement of the left leg.

1. Lie flat on the back and raise the left knee toward the chest, holding it with both hands. Angle the knee until it is over the navel. Tension occurs in the lower left abdomen.

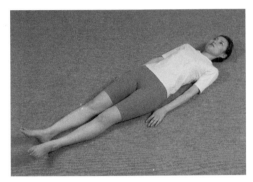

Lie flat on the back.

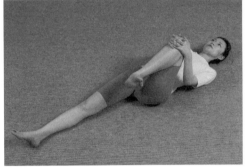

Raise the left knee toward the chest, holding it with both hands. Angle the knee until it is over the navel. Turn the foot outward. Increase the tension by trying to push the knee away from the body.

2. Turn the foot outward and hold its position. Increase the tension by trying to push the knee away from the body using leg force while pulling the knee tighter toward the navel with the hands and arms.

3. Release the hands and extend the leg quickly and drop it on the floor. Suddenly loosening the tension in the left lower abdomen activates the functions of the colon and rectum.

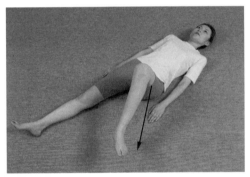

Release the hands and extend the leg quickly and drop it on the floor.

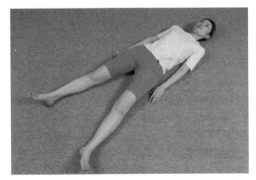

Suddenly loosening the tension in the left lower abdomen activates the function of the colon and rectum.

OBESITY

■ GENERAL REMARKS

The cause of obesity, a condition characterized by excessive body fat, is usually attributed to food intake that exceeds the amount the body needs for metabolic change and movement. The surplus energy is stored in the body as fat. Average height-weight ratios, body fat ratios, etc., are used as standards to determine obesity.

Obesity is a concern for many men and women regarding appearance. In addition, obesity can lead to a variety of illnesses. Weight-reducing methods, such as various diets and exercises, abound throughout the world.

■ SEITAI POINT OF VIEW

Firstly, Seitai does not support the idea that an individual be compared to some average weight ratio. To be deemed overweight or under-weight on numerical values alone does not necessarily indicate bodily disorder. On the contrary, more harm can be done when attempting to forcefully conform to some objective average ratio. In addition, as there are many slim people who consume large quantities of food, obesity cannot be explained only in terms of the relationship between energy produced by food intake and energy consumed.

From the Seitai point of view, when the pelvis of an individual opens and shifts down, the individual's constitution tends toward easily becoming overweight. Many mothers, as a result of not observing the rest period after child delivery as prescribed by Seitai, have pelvic trouble and become overweight. This may be a reason why many women are overweight in countries where it is customary to start walking soon after child delivery.

If the pelvis returns to its normal condition, the body weight also reverts to what is suitable for the individual.

■ SELF-TREATMENT

The iliac bone exercise (see pp. 123–125) and pelvic exercise are effective in restoring the dropped and laterally opened pelvis to its normal condition. Moreover, the breastbone exercise (see pp. 115–118) is recommended in cases where obesity is caused by pelvic disorder attributable to lung trouble. This exercise recovers the mobility of the shoulder blades and gathers them toward the central vertical axis of the body. The pelvis, which works together with the shoulder blades, also tightens and closes inward. As a result, the problem of obesity is resolved.

The above exercises are equally effective for men, and for women who have not delivered a child.

PELVIC EXERCISE

1. Lie on the back, raise the knees, and draw the heels near the buttocks.

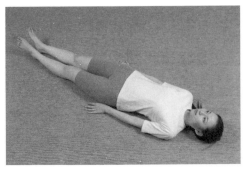

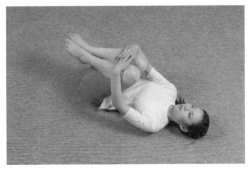

Lie on the back.

Raise the knees and draw the heels near the buttocks.

2. Open the knees widely and keep the soles of the feet about one fist-width apart.

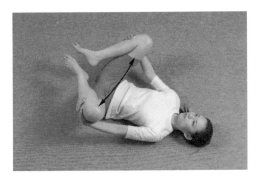

Open the knees widely and keep the soles of the feet about one fist-width apart.

3. Extend the lower legs while maintaining the angle of the upper legs. Push the heels out to stretch the Achilles tendons and turn the feet inward. Extend the left and right heels alternately. Feel the stretching along the back of the thighs, calves, and Achilles tendons.

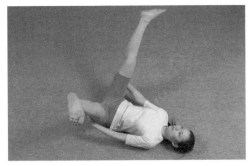

Extend the lower legs while maintaining the angle of the upper legs. Push the heels out to stretch the Achilles tendons and turn the feet inward.

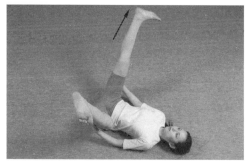 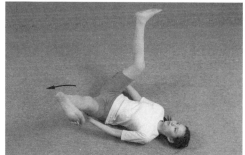

Extend the left and right heels alternately.

4. Slowly lower the opened legs and hold the heels at a height of about 10cm while stretching out the heels. Lower the legs slowly onto the floor.

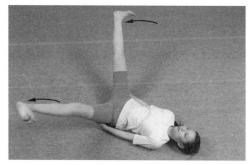 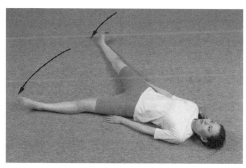

Slowly lower the opened legs.

Lower the legs slowly onto the floor.

NOTE: The feet should be turned inward until the exercise is completed, if possible. Pregnant women, and women in a postnatal period, should not perform this exercise.

Chapter 7

WOMEN'S AILMENTS

CYSTITIS (INFLAMMATION OF THE BLADDER)

■ **GENERAL REMARKS**

Cystitis, inflammation or infection of the urinary bladder caused by such bacteria as coliform bacillus, begins in the urinary system.

Cystitis more commonly occurs when the body's immune system becomes weak. Women generally suffer from cystitis more easily, since the urinary tract in women is shorter than that in men. The main symptoms of cystitis are:

(1) Urinating with abnormal frequency.

(2) The feeling that the bladder does not completely empty.

(3) Pain when urinating.

(4) Bloody or opaque urine.

■ **SEITAI POINT OF VIEW**

The cause of cystitis, other than that attributed to bacteria, is insufficient filtration of body waste due to dysfunction in the kidneys caused by fatigue. As a result of the weakening of the kidneys, the urine becomes too acidic and harmful to the bladder, leaving the bladder more vulnerable to infection. As the bladder loses its ability to function efficiently, the urine is not completely discharged upon urinating.

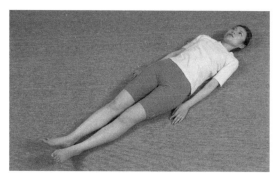
Lie on the back.

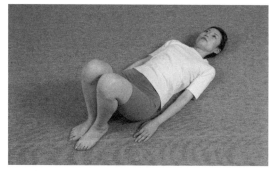
Raise both knees while pulling the heels to the buttocks.

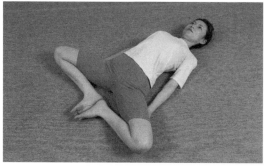
Join the soles of the feet and let the bent legs fall naturally out to their widest position.

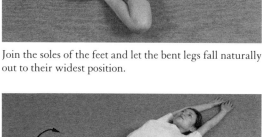
Extend both arms overhead, and sway the knees left and right very slightly and slowly.

The remaining urine adversely affects the bladder allowing bacteria to more easily multiply and accumulate.

The function of the kidneys and bladder is related to T10, L3, and L5. Furthermore, the function of T4 and T5, related to the control of perspiration, is also associated with bladder inflammation. For example, body waste accumulates in an individual who has difficulty sweating sufficiently during the summer. As a result, the accumulated waste becomes a burden on the kidneys and causes inflammation of the bladder.

■ SELF-TREATMENT

When the pain of cystitis is acute, apply a hot moist towel over the area of the bladder where the pain is most severe. The hot moist towel method is normally repeated every 8 hours. However, in the case of acute pain, repeat the second hot towel treatment 4 hours after the first one. Start the third treatment 6 hours after the second one and the next one 8 hours after the third one. The 2-hour interval must be observed, since the 4–6–8-hour interval is based on the internal cycle of changes in the body.

Do the physical exercise for L5, which helps to recover the function of the kidneys (and bladder) and enhances the body's ability to expel urine. In addition, the bladder builds resistance to cystitis as the bacteria entering the body are excreted in the urine.

EXERCISE FOR L5

Lie on the back and raise both knees while pulling the heels to the buttocks. Join the soles of the feet and let the bent legs fall naturally out to their widest position. Slightly arch the lumbar region to bring tension to the base of the lumbar vertebra L5. Holding this posture, sway the knees left and right very slightly and slowly, ensuring to keep the axis of the movement in L5. When the exercise is done properly, tension will build in L5.

MENSTRUAL PAIN

■ GENERAL REMARKS

The main symptoms of menstrual pain, such as abdominal pain, lower back pain, headaches, nausea, etc., vary according to the individual. For some women, the associated discomfort becomes serious enough to disrupt daily activities, even the ability to leave home. In such cases, it is recommendable to consult with a specialist, as this could indicate serious internal problems.

■ SEITAI POINT OF VIEW

The cause of menstrual pain originates in L4. The source of abnormality in L4 varies by individual, and can include trouble in the stomach, the digestive system, the urinary system, the respiratory system, the nervous system, abnormal secretion of hormones, gynecological problems, or an injury to the pelvis.

Menstrual bleeding begins with the relaxation of the pelvis. When the mobility of L4 is restricted, however, the relaxation of the left and right sides of the pelvis does not proceed symmetrically. Such imbalance in the pelvis places excessive strain on the lumbar area, creating the menstrual pain.

■ SELF-TREATMENT

A fundamental treatment is to do the illiac bone exercise (see pp. 123–125) to recover the mobility of L4 and ease the movement of the pelvis. Furthermore, it is recommendable to do the pubic bone exercise (see pp. 135–137) to tighten the pelvis. Taking a footbath regularly improves the body's circulation and helps to alleviate menstrual pain.

To prevent menstrual pain, it is recommendable to do the preventive exercise for menstrual pain (see below) daily before the menstrual cycle begins, once in the morning and again before going to bed. In the event of pain, apply the hot moist towel method to the area of L4 after doing the exercise. If the abdominal pain is acute, apply the hot moist towel method directly to the aching area.

EXERCISE FOR THE PREVENTION OF MENSTRUAL PAIN

Lie on the back. Raise the knees while pulling the heels toward the buttocks until the soles of the feet rest comfortably on the floor. Lean the bent legs together slowly to the left and right several times. Lean only the legs, being careful to avoid twisting the upper half of the body or raising it from the floor.

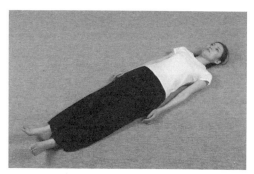

Lie on the back.

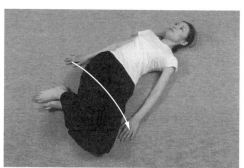

Raise the knees while pulling the heels toward the buttocks. Lean the bent legs together slowly to the left and right several times.

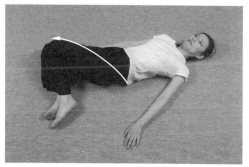

Lean only the legs, being careful to avoid twisting the upper half of the body or raising it from the floor.

GALLSTONES

■ GENERAL REMARKS

Women suffer from cholelithiasis, the formation of gallstones, about twice as much as men. When eating, bile is secreted from the gallbladder to digest fats. The bile is carried from the gallbladder to the upper small intestine (duodenum) through the common bile duct. If the bile in the gallbladder becomes chemically unbalanced or stagnates in the gallbladder, it can harden into particles that can eventually grow into gallstones. Gallstones often go undetected until a steady ache or pain becomes present in the upper-middle or upper-right abdomen.

■ SEITAI POINT OF VIEW

The medical world cites a diet high in fat (especially animal fat) and sugar as increasing the risk of gallstones. However, from the Seitai point of view, the main cause of the problem is mental stress, which causes the secretion of bile to deteriorate. The symptoms of gallstones occur most often when the individual suffers from anxiety or is deprived of sleep for a long time.

■ SELF-TREATMENT

As a fundamental treatment, it is necessary to eliminate mental stress and to obtain sufficient sleep.

To ease the pain of gallstones, it is necessary to normalize the function of the gallbladder by recovering the mobility of T9, the related vertebra. The combined exercise (see pp. 127–129) is effective for this purpose. When the pain is acute, it may seem totally impossible to do the exercise, but the area stiffened due to the pain will gradually relax and the pain will subside. When the body is stretched to the left or right, more pain may occur at a specific point. The efficacy of the exercise is increased when more stimulus is applied to the specific point.

The hot moist towel method is usually applied to the painful point on the abdomen after completing the exercise, but if the pain is severe, apply the hot moist towel method before doing the exercise to ease the pain.

MENOPAUSAL DISORDERS

■ GENERAL REMARKS

The symptoms of menopausal disorders generally begin to appear in women aged 40 to 50 before, during, and after menopause. Menopause occurs when the production of the female hormones estrogen and progesterone decreases. The main symptoms of menopausal disorders include headaches, stiff shoulders, hot flushes, etc., and women can suffer from several symptoms simultaneously. The body parts affected and the type of discomfort differ according to the individual, who is also affected by environmental changes, such as the weather, and mental stress.

■ SEITAI POINT OF VIEW

All women experience menopause and the decrease in production of female hormones as they grow older. The source of menopausal disorder is the body itself, which is incapable of adapting to changes associated with menopause. To be precise, the body is not able to change in accordance with the decreased production of female hormones (associated with L4) that causes a variety of problems, such as hot flushes (associated with T5).

A stiff body tends to show drastic and prolonged reactions to every internal and external change, such as menopause, or the change of seasons, and so on. The body's ability to adapt to such changes is determined by its elasticity. By relaxing a stiff body, it is possible to pass through menopause without encountering serious problems.

■ SELF-TREATMENT

Rather than attempting to alleviate every symptom of menopausal disorders, Seitai places emphasis on relaxing the body's tendency to stiffen, which is the fundamental cause of the problems. The Seitai physical exercise to loosen the spinal column (see pp. 52–53) is effective for this purpose.

When the symptoms of menopausal disorders are serious, it is sometimes difficult to feel that the entire body is being relaxed with this exercise, since stiffness remains in the arms, legs, waist, among other areas. By continuing the exercise, though, flexibility gradually appears, which produces a positive effect on the whole body.

It is recommendable to apply the hot moist towel method to the area where stiffness and discomfort are experienced. In particular, various symptoms are temporarily relieved if the towel is applied to the chest, which has weakened as a result of mental stress and other adverse influences.

SENSITIVITY TO COLD

■ GENERAL REMARKS

Women suffer from sensitivity to cold more than men. The main symptom is cold hands and feet. When the symptom is serious, the coldness of the limbs cannot be eradicated no matter what degree of heat is applied, and the ability to sleep is interrupted.

■ SEITAI POINT OF VIEW

The body attempts to maintain a constant body temperature. Therefore, a healthy body keeps a constant temperature even if the air temperature rises or falls. Sensitivity to cold occurs when the body is unable to keep the temperature of its extremities constant. This is the result of a disorder in the body's temperature adjusting function associated with T4 and T5.

Moreover, in response to excessive stimulus, the body becomes stiff in an attempt to defend itself. Since the defense response to coldness is excessive in the body of the individual who is sensitive to cold, the body rapidly stiffens in response to even a slight drop in temperature. Hence, the individual falls into a vicious cycle in which the circulation of body fluid deteriorates as a result of body stiffness and the symptoms of coldness escalate because of the weakened circulation.

■ SELF-TREATMENT

Of prime importance is to perspire sufficiently during the hot summer months in order to develop a body that is capable of flexibly adjusting to climatic changes. Perspiration promotes metabolism as well as blood and lymph circulation. As a result, the body relaxes and body fluids are able to flow unobstructed through the entire body throughout the year, enhancing the body's ability to maintain a constant temperature. Furthermore, the transmission of nerve impulses becomes smooth as the body relaxes and its ability to adapt to environmental changes normalizes.

If sleeping becomes difficult because of severe coldness in the extremities, taking a footbath before going to bed is recommended. Though only the feet are soaked to the middle of the ankle, the footbath helps to improve the circulation in the feet as well as the hands.

The breastbone exercise (see p. 115–118), which strengthens the respiratory system, is also effective, though doing this exercise is difficult for individuals with sensitivity to cold, as they generally have weaker lungs. That being said, doing the exercise eventually becomes easier and the symptoms of coldness will diminish. The lymphatic exercise (see pp. 118–123) and C-shape exercise (see pp. 138–139) are also effective.

Chapter 8

CHILDREN'S AILMENTS

TONSILLITIS

■ GENERAL REMARKS

Tonsillitis, an infection and inflammation of the tonsils, is usually caused by group A beta-hemolytic streptococcus bacteria. Preschool and school-aged children are the most common sufferers of tonsillitis. The signs and symptoms of tonsillitis include severe sore throat, difficulty in swallowing, headache, fever and chills, and tender cervical lymph nodes.

There are three forms of tonsillitis: acute, with a rapid onset of significant symptoms; subacute, with a slow onset of less obvious symptoms; and chronic, with intermittent symptoms that persist over time.

■ SEITAI POINT OF VIEW

Although bacteria and viruses are constantly present in the air, some individuals become easily infected while others do not. This would indicate that the cause of an infectious disease cannot be attributed solely to the existence of bacteria, and that the homeostatic condition of the individual must also be taken into consideration.

The main cause of tonsillitis is dysfunction in the urinary organs (kidneys), which affects the tonsils. This is apparent from the high incidence of chronic kidney disease sufferers that contract tonsillitis.

Observing the body of individuals with tonsillitis, L3, T5, and

T10 which relate to the kidneys, lack vitality and some abnormality also appears in C5 and C6.

In the past, surgery to remove tonsils was once the standard treatment for tonsillitis. However, the tonsils, which help prevent harmful bacteria and viruses that could cause more serious infections from entering the body, comprise an important part of the body's immune system. Inflammation is one of the body's natural reactions to fight off bacteria and viruses. From this point of view, to remove the tonsils is to remove a part of the body's immune system. It is questionable whether surgery has been the most appropriate treatment for tonsillitis.

■ SELF-TREATMENT

To ease acute symptoms of tonsillitis, apply the hot moist towel method directly onto the aching area. In the case of chronic tonsillitis, which Seitai believes must be related to kidney dysfunction and the stagnation of body waste, it is recommendable to take the footbath twice a day, once in the morning and again in the evening.

TYMPANITIS

■ GENERAL REMARKS

Tympanitis (also called *otitis media*), or inflammation in the middle ear, is caused by bacteria and occurs mostly in infants and young children. Acute tympanitis involves a high fever and severe ear pain. The condition can deteriorate and become chronic if matter exudes and accumulates in the ear.

From the medical perspective, tympanitis does not develop from bacteria directly entering the ear, but rather from respiratory infection, such as a cold, whereby bacteria passes through the auditory tube connecting the back of the nose to the middle ear.

■ SEITAI POINT OF VIEW

Diseases in the nose and ears, such as tympanitis, are very often attributed to overeating. Overeating raises T6, related to the function of the stomach, and adheres it to T5. This has an effect on C4, which is related to the nose. The symptoms start from blockage in the nose and this in turn affects the ear, manifesting as tympanitis. However, some children have recently suffered from this condition because of neurological factors, such as mental stress, making it more difficult to determine the specific source of the disease.

Children sometimes begin to cry suddenly during the night because of pain associated with tympanitis. When the acute pain is severe and difficult to endure, apply the hot moist towel method to the back of the head, from the upper neck to C4.

For chronic tympanitis, it is recommendable to first do the Seitai exercise to loosen the spinal column (see pp. 52–53) in order to relax the whole body and then the combined exercise (see pp. 127–129) to enhance the function of the digestive organs. These exercises restore the proper function of T5 and T6 and alleviate the discomfort of tympanitis. The fundamental treatment of tympanitis, however, is to eliminate the habit of overeating.

ASTHMA

■ GENERAL REMARKS

The most common form of asthma, a chronic condition that occurs when the main air passages of the lungs (bronchial tubes) become inflamed, is bronchial asthma. The symptoms of asthma include wheezing, coughing, production of excess mucus, and difficulty breathing. The symptoms can manifest as a violent fit or asthma attack, which, in the worst cases, can be life-threatening. Generally, the cause of asthma is thought to be some form of allergy.

■ SEITAI POINT OF VIEW

Not all allergy sufferers have asthma, meaning that the cause of asthma is some reason other than an allergy. The following are the three main reasons of the occurrence of asthma from the viewpoint of Seitai:

(1) A mental disorder manifests in the form of an asthma attack. Most infants and youths with asthma are under constant high mental stress. The desire to escape from the excessive stress causes asthma.

(2) The function of the respiratory system is naturally weak.

(3) The thorax is stiff due to overeating. Coughing develops to release the stress, but the cough progresses to asthma-like symptoms.

■ SELF-TREATMENT

When the cause of asthma is thought to be attributed to mental stress or overeating, such causes must be removed. The cooperation of family members is essential.

If the asthma is caused by weakness of the respiratory system, a fundamental change in bodily function is required. It is most effective to activate the cutaneous respiration of the entire body by perspiring sufficiently in summer. The activated cutaneous respiration lightens the burden of the entire respiratory system.

The deep breathing method (see pp. 114–115) also enhances the function of the respiratory system.

The C-shape exercise (see pp. 138–139), the breastbone exercise (see pp. 115–118) and the lymphatic exercise (see pp. 118–123) are effective for asthma sufferers. Applying the hot moist towel method around the bronchus area of the upper chest after doing the exercises produces added benefits. Furthermore, the hot moist towel method to the upper chest eases an asthma attack and relaxes breathing.

ATOPIC DERMATITIS

■ GENERAL REMARKS

Although atopic dermatitis usually appears in infants and becomes less of a problem in adulthood, recently the disease has become increasingly common in adults. At the outset of atopic dermatitis, the skin is red, moist, and rough. It subsequently becomes dry, encrusted, and itchy. Scratching the affected area breaks open the skin, fluid secretes to the surface, and the cycle of drying, itching, and scratching repeats again and again. Generally, allergies are regarded as the cause of atopic dermatitis.

■ SEITAI POINT OF VIEW

As not all allergy sufferers have asthma, not all allergy sufferers have atopic dermatitis. This indicates that the cause of the problem exists in the individual body.

Observing the body of individuals with atopic dermatitis, the function of the respiratory system is dull and, for this reason, the body is not able to adapt itself to changing seasons or mental stress. The same reason explains why the symptoms appear or become serious when seasons change, especially from winter to spring, and from summer to fall. In the case of adults, it is characteristic that L4, which typically relaxes in spring, remains stiff. As a result, the body is unable to adapt to the change of season. It should also be noted that all skin problems are closely related to mental factors, such as anxiety, and the respiratory system.

■ SELF-TREATMENT

It is recommendable to do the breastbone exercise (see pp. 115–118), which activates the function of the respiratory system. The skin and lungs relate to each other by means of cutaneous respiration. Symptoms of skin problems appear easily when the respiratory system is weakened. When atopic dermatitis appears, cutaneous respiration is obstructed by skin inflammation. This becomes a serious burden on the lungs and makes them less flexible.

The breastbone exercise improves the function of the lungs. The exercise normalizes the position of the scapulas, raises the collarbone, and relaxes the thorax. The exercise should be done 3 times daily— in the morning, at noon, and at night.

It is also beneficial to apply the hot moist towel method directly on the inflamed skin. The heat and the humidity of the towel promote circulation and cause the pores to open. As body waste is excreted from the opened pores, the symptoms may seem to deteriorate, temporarily, before they improve.

Chapter 9

SEITAI EXERCISES

DEEP BREATHING METHOD—*SHINSOKU-HO*

1. Lie on the back. Place one hand on the upper tanden and the other on the lower tanden and assess the condition of each. In a normal state, the upper tanden is relaxed and flexible and the lower tanden is firm and strong.

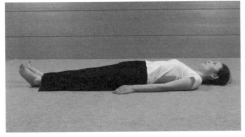

Lie on the back.

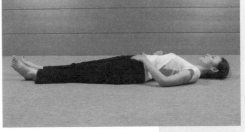

Place one hand on the upper tanden and the other on the lower tanden.

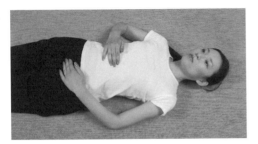

Assess the condition of each tanden.

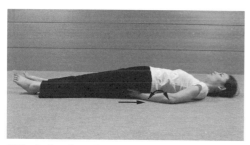

Slide the hands under the hips as if to grab the buttocks.

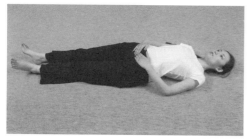

Place both hands on the lower tanden and lightly close the eyes.

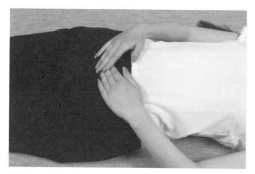

Without inhaling, expand only the lower abdomen about 60–70%.

2. Slide the hands under the hips as if to grab the buttocks. Pull the hands up along the buttocks to raise the hips and emphasize the arch of the lumbar area. Hold this position.

3. Place both hands on the lower tanden and lightly close the eyes. Inhale deeply and exhale completely.

4. Without inhaling, expand only the lower abdomen about 60–70%. Feel the lower tanden strengthen. Holding the tension in the lower abdomen, take shallow breaths using only the chest, but avoid straining the upper abdomen.

5. Continue such breathing for approximately 30 seconds. Inhale deeply and open the right eye first to prevent excessive stimulus to the body on exhaling and then the left eye. It is best to gradually extend the duration of the shinsoku-ho training to about 3 minutes.

Upper tanden: Vital point on the central vertical axis of the abdomen located 3-finger widths below the lowest point of the sternum.

Lower tanden: Vital point on the central vertical axis of the abdomen located 3-finger widths above the pubic bone.

BREASTBONE (STERNUM) EXERCISE

■ EFFECTS

• Eases stiffness in the shoulders and fatigue in the arms.
• Activates the function of the respiratory system.

The shoulders consist of three bones—the humerus (upper arm bone), scapula (shoulder blade), and clavicle (collarbone)—connected by joints. When muscle tension around the shoulders is caused by shoulder stiffness, for example, the thorax will be stiff, since the shoulder blades slide laterally away from the central vertical axis and the ribs also shift from the center due to the lower position of the clavicles. This stiffness inhibits deep breathing. The effect of this exercise is to return the opened and stiff thorax and related parts to their normal position.

1. Stand on your knees and interlace your fingers as shown in the picture. Leave the thumbs freely open.

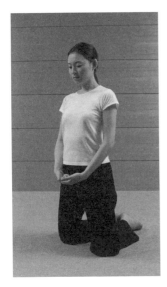

Stand on your knees and interlace your fingers.

2. Bend your interlaced fingers at the second joint to hitch the fingers to one another. Do not cross your fingers. If the shoulder blades have slid away from the center and/or the pectoralis major muscles are stiff, interlacing the fingers as indicated is difficult.

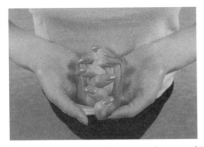 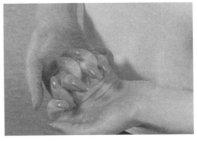

Bend your interlaced fingers at the second joint to hitch the fingers to one another.

3. Stretch the extended arms lightly and slowly over the head. This movement helps to raise lower positioned ribs.

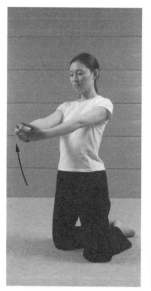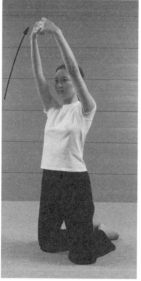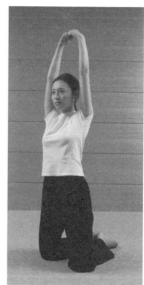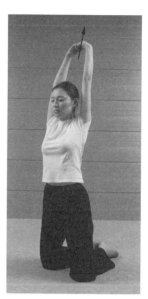

Stretch the extended arms lightly and slowly over the head.

4. Bring the arms down behind the head while bending the elbows, and place the interlocked hands on the back of the head. While holding this position, extend the elbows backward and hold out the chest.

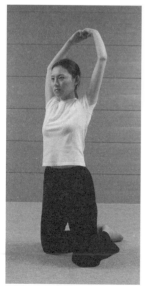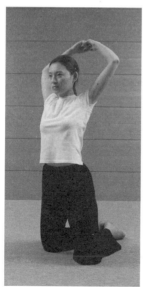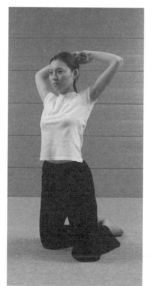

Bring the arms down behind the head while bending the elbows, and place the interlocked hands on the back of the head.

5. With the support of the head, extend the elbows further back to move the shoulder blades toward the center. This movement helps to raise the dropped clavicles.

6. Alternately incline each elbow downward and upward slowly while extending the elbows back. To stretch the pectoralis major muscles easily, pull the upper positioned elbow back a little further than the opposite elbow.

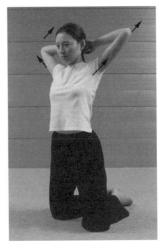

With the support of the head, extend the elbows further back.

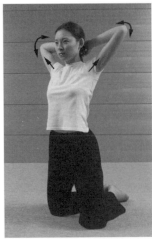

Alternately incline each elbow downward and upward slowly.

LYMPHATIC EXERCISE A (BASIC)

■ **EFFECTS**

• Improves lymph circulation.
• Boosts the immune system.

The functions of the lymph fluid circulation include the elimination of body waste. In addition, the lymph nodes, generally called "lymph glands," act as a kind of filter to eliminate bacteria and viruses by producing white blood cells linked to the immune system.

Lymphatic exercises activate the function of the lymph nodes and improve lymph circulation throughout the body by stretching the armpits, an area where lymph nodes are concentrated, and by raising the position of the ribs to ease intercostal stiffness.

1. Stand on the knees, interlace the fingers of both hands as shown in the picture, turn the palms down, and extend the arms lightly. If it is difficult to interlace the fingers, hold the wrist as indicated.

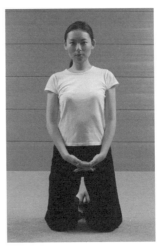

Stand on the knees, interlace the fingers of both hands.

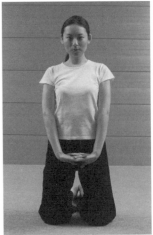

Turn the palms down.

2. Raise the extended arms over the head while holding the hands together. When the hands are directly above the head, stretch them lightly upward.

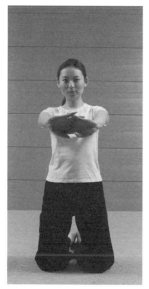 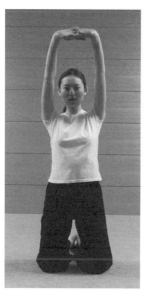 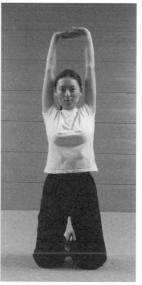

Extend the arms lightly.

Raise the extended arms over the head while holding the hands together.

When the hands are directly above the head, stretch them lightly upward.

3. Incline the body a little toward the right and stretch the left armpit and intercostal area by stretching the arms further

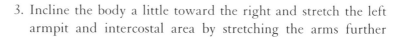

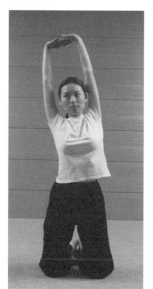 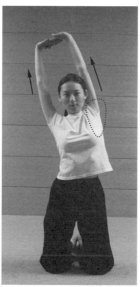 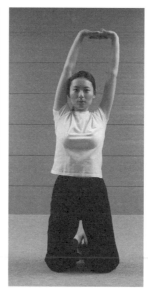 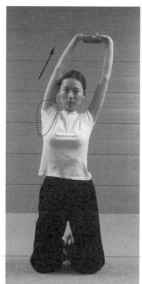

Incline the body a little toward the right and stretch the left armpit and intercostal area by stretching the arms further upward.

upward. Hold this position for 2–3 breaths. Repeat the movement for the opposite side.

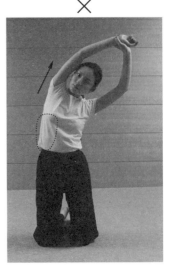

NOTE: Inclining the body too much will stretch the side of the body instead of the ribs. This will render the exercise ineffective.

Inclining the body too much will stretch the side of the body instead of the ribs.

LYMPHATIC EXERCISE B (TWISTING)

■ **EFFECTS**

• Improves lymph circulation.
• Boosts the immune system.

This exercise improves the mobility of the ribs eased by the basic lymphatic exercise. The basic exercise raises the ribs on both sides of the body. Adding to that, this exercise helps to stretch the ribs in the front and the back.

1. Stand on the knees and hold the right wrist with the left hand in front of the body.

2. Bend the right elbow and position it alongside the body. While lowering the right shoulder, pull the right arm toward the left side until the right elbow is near the navel. Ensure the elbow is close to the body.

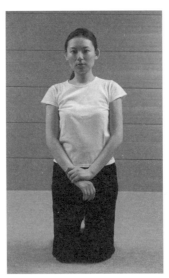

Stand on the knees and hold the right wrist with the left hand in front of the body.

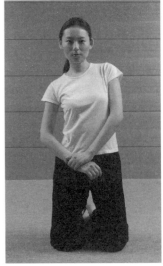

Bend the right elbow and position it alongside the body.

3. With the left hand, pull the right arm obliquely upward. This movement helps to stretch the upper body upward while twisting it at the same time. Be sure to feel that the back ribs are stretched. Repeat the procedure on the left side.

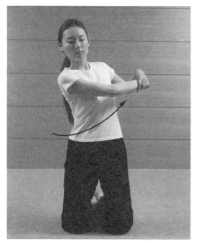 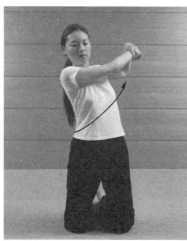 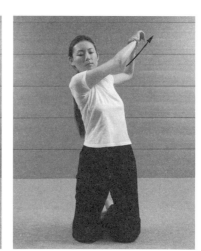

While lowering the right shoulder, pull the right arm toward the left side until the right elbow is near the navel.

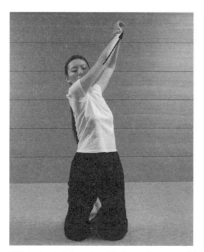 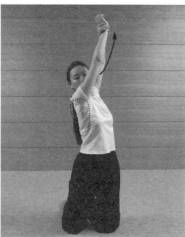

With the left hand, pull the right arm obliquely upward.

LYMPHATIC EXERCISE C (LYING)

■ **EFFECTS**

• Improves lymph circulation.
• Boosts the immune system.

People having trouble moving the body freely will find this exercise relatively easy, since it can be done while lying on the back. This exercise lessens fatigue only if done before going to bed or after waking. This exercise is also useful to confirm that the movements in the basic and twisting lymphatic exercises are being done correctly.

1. Lie on the back, clasp the hands as in the basic exercise, turn the palms down, and stretch the arms lightly.

2. Slowly raise the extended arms upward.

3. While raising the arms, a point is reached where they cannot easily be raised further. At this point, slightly incline the upper body while stretching the arms as in the basic exercise.

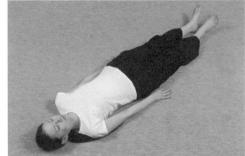

Lie on the back.

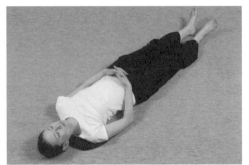

Clasp the hands as in the basic exercise.

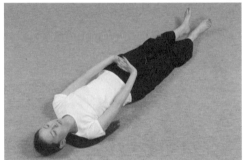

Turn the palms down.

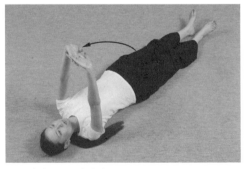

Stretch the arms lightly.

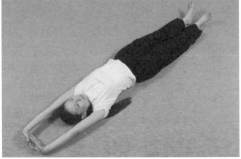

Slowly raise the extended arms upward, and slightly incline the upper body.

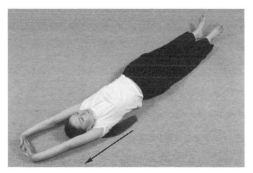

Slightly incline the upper body. Extend the arms further over the head to stretch the armpits and intercostal areas.

4. Extend the arms further over the head to stretch the armpits and intercostal areas. Hold the position for 2–3 breaths and relax the arms. Repeat the movement on the opposite side.

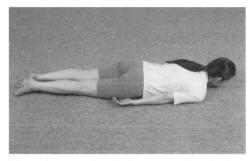

Lie on the stomach with the arms at the sides, legs together, toes in, and heels out.

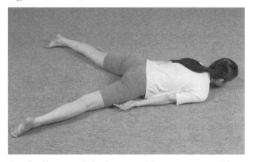

Gradually spread the legs as wide apart as possible.

ILIAC BONE EXERCISE (1)

CAUTIONARY NOTE: Pregnant women should avoid doing this exercise.

■ EFFECTS

• Activates the function of the respiratory system.
• Relieves backache.

The iliac is a vital bone in our body since it is related to the lower back, the respiratory system, the urinary system, the cervical vertebrae, and the brain. Improving the mobility of the iliac bone with this exercise affects all of the related parts. This exercise works especially well for improving the function of the respiratory system. Furthermore, this exercise exerts pressure on each lumbar vertebra in such a way as to restore them to their normal position.

1. Lie on the stomach with the arms at the sides, legs together, toes in, and heels out. Gradually spread the legs as wide apart as possible.

2. Lift the lower legs to join the soles of the feet together while keeping the legs apart. Spread the knees apart as far as possible.

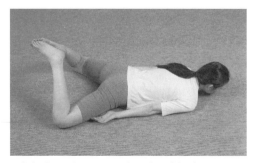

Lift the lower legs to join the soles of the feet together while keeping the legs apart.

3. Pull the heels of the feet as close to the buttocks as possible while keeping the soles of the feet flat together.

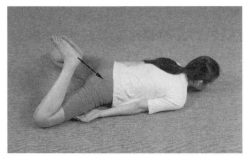

Pull the heels of the feet as close to the buttocks as possible.

4. Angle the toes up toward the ceiling and hold the position for 2–3 breaths.

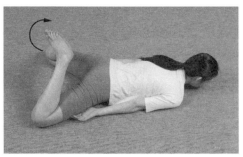

Angle the toes up toward the ceiling and hold the position for 2–3 breaths.

ILIAC BONE EXERCISE (2)

CAUTIONARY NOTE: Pregnant women should avoid doing this exercise.

■ EFFECTS

• Activates the function of the respiratory system.
• Strengthens the lower back.

The main purpose of the iliac bone exercise is to return the angle of the iliac bone to normal by concentrating the strength of the lower legs and hip joints into the iliac bone. To increase the effectiveness of this exercise, stretch the arms out laterally and over the head as shown in the picture.

1. Complete the exercise following the instructions for Iliac bone exercise 1.

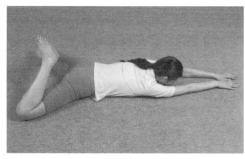

Gradually slide the arms out from alongside the body and up over the head.

2. While holding the position, gradually slide the arms out from alongside the body and up over the head. Stretch the arms out while keeping the tension concentrated in the iliac bone.

ILIAC BONE EXERCISE (3)

CAUTIONARY NOTE: Pregnant women should avoid doing this exercise.

■ **EFFECTS**

- Activates the function of the respiratory system.
- Strengthens the lower back.

In this exercise, concentrate the strength of the lower legs and upper body into the iliac bone. Once familiar with this exercise, it will be possible to concentrate strength into abnormalities in the iliac bone, such as pain or fatigue, by freely using the strength of the lower legs and upper body.

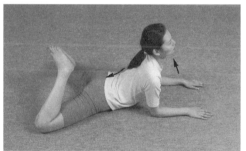

Lift the upper body with the support of the arms.

1. Complete the exercise following the instructions for Iliac bone exercise 2.

2. While holding the final position, lift the upper body with the support of the arms. Keep the strength of the upper body concentrated into the iliac bone while lifting the upper body.

LOWER BACK EXERCISE

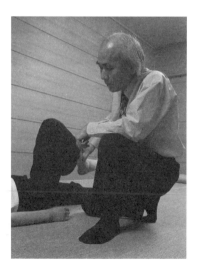

■ **EFFECTS**

- Eases or prevents backache.

When experiencing a backache, such as acute lower back pain, the lower back muscles and the lumbar spine itself are stiff. This exercise helps to quickly relieve the pain by easing the stiffness. If intense pain hampers leg movement, bend the knees only slightly and initially rotate the legs in small circles. Then, gradually increase the size of the circular rotation and stretch the legs to ease the pain in order to relax the lower back area. Performing this exercise daily helps to prevent backache.

1. Lie on the back with the arms at the sides and slightly lift the legs. Stretch your Achilles tendons by pushing the heels out.

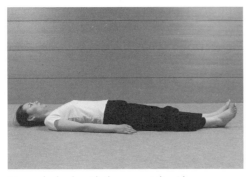 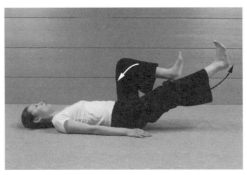

Lie on the back with the arms at the sides.

Slightly lift the legs. Stretch your Achilles tendons by pushing the heels out.

2. Alternately, slowly stretch out one leg from the heel while bringing the knee of the other leg up and over the abdomen, as though back-pedaling on a bicycle.

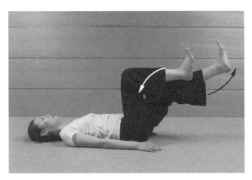 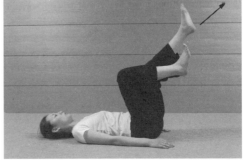

Alternately, slowly stretch out one leg from the heel while bringing the knee of the other leg up and over the abdomen.

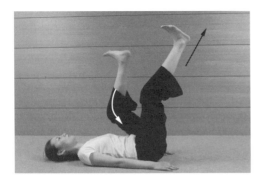

3. Repeat step 2 while very gradually increasing the angle of the legs from the horizontal position until the legs are fully upright and perpendicular to the floor. At this point, continue the backward pedaling movement and start to gradually work back to the horizontal position. Repeat the entire movement twice.

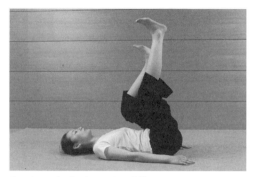

Continue the backward pedaling movement.

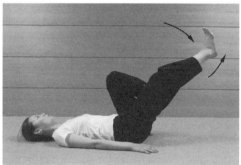

Start to gradually work back to the horizontal position.

Experiencing discomfort with the legs at a certain angle indicates a problem in the lower back corresponding to the angle of incidence. To increase the effectiveness of this exercise, move the legs especially slowly at the angle where the greatest tension is felt in the lower back.

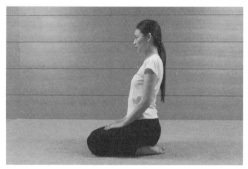

Squat on the floor.

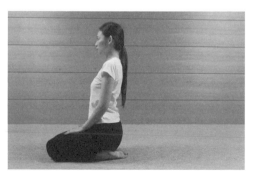

Keep the lower legs tucked under the upper legs and buttocks.

COMBINED EXERCISE (OVEREATING AND LYMPH)

■ EFFECTS

• Strengthens the immune system.
• Recovers the function of the digestive system.

This exercise is a combination of the lymphatic exercise and overeating exercise. These exercises are effective in strengthening the immune system and recovering the function of the digestive system, respectively. Combining the two exercises generates synergistic effects owing to their close connection.

1. Squat on the floor as shown in the picture. Keep the lower legs tucked under the upper legs and buttocks.

2. Slowly bring the upper body down backward with the support of the arms.

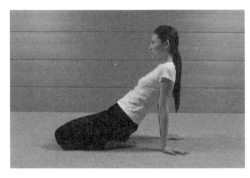

Slowly bring the upper body down backward with the support of the arms.

3. Keep the knees and the back on the floor. To ease physical discomfort, slowly open and close the knees slightly, or bring the knees together and gently shift them left and right. This movement helps to stretch the front of the thighs and relax the stiffened part of the spine obstructing the movement.

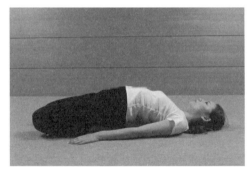

Keep the knees and the back on the floor.

4. Bring the hands over the abdomen, interlock the fingers, and turn the palms toward the feet.

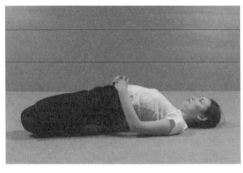 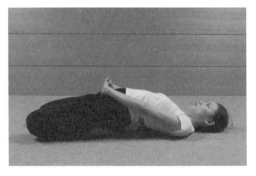

Bring the hands over the abdomen, interlock the fingers.

Turn the palms toward the feet.

5. Raise the extended arms out and up over the head.

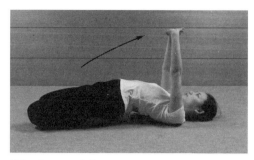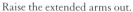

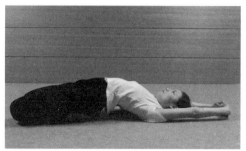

Raise the extended arms out.

Raise them up over the head.

6. Keeping the arms straight, incline the body a little and stretch the arms obliquely upward to stretch the armpit and ribs. Hold the position for 2–3 breaths. Repeat the movement twice on each side.

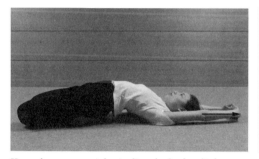

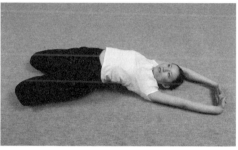

Keep the arms straight, incline the body a little.

Stretch the arms obliquely upward to stretch the armpit and ribs.

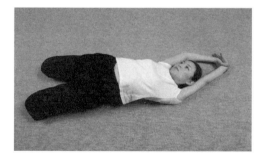

Repeat the movement twice on each side.

NOTE: Keep the knees pressed to the floor as much as possible.

L-SHAPE EXERCISE (1)

■ EFFECTS

• Activates the function of the respiratory system and kidneys.
• Improves the mobility of the iliac bones and ischiatic bones.

The back thigh muscle, the biceps femoris, is related to the iliac bones. Relieving the stiffness of the biceps femoris by means of this exercise relaxes the related iliac bones.

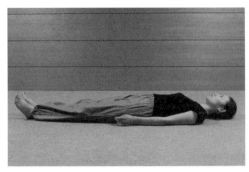
Lie on the back.

1. Lie on the back.

2. Gradually lift the bent legs up toward the abdomen, stopping just before the point where the lower back lifts from the floor.

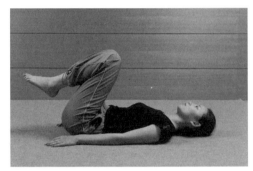
Gradually lift the bent legs up toward the abdomen.

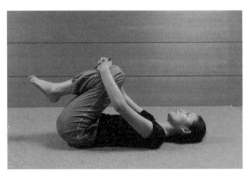
Stop just before the point where the lower back lifts from the floor.

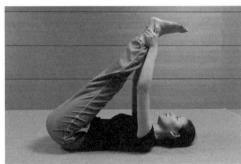
Stretch out the legs and push the heels outward to stretch the Achilles tendons.

3. Stretch out the legs and push the heels outward to stretch the Achilles tendons. Hold the legs wherever possible, ideally the ankles, with the hands.

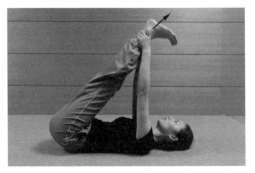
Hold the legs wherever possible, ideally the ankles, with the hands.

4. Alternately, push the heels further outward with slow, small movements. This movement helps to stretch the Achilles tendons, the backs of the knees, and the biceps femoris.

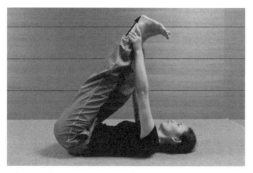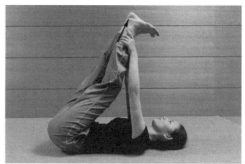

Alternately, push the heels further outward with slow, small movements.

NOTE: This exercise is ineffective if the knees are bent excessively.

L-SHAPE EXERCISE (2)

■ **EFFECTS**

• Activates the functions of the respiratory system and kidneys.
• Improves the mobility of the iliac bones and ischiatic bones.

This exercise is designed for those who have trouble doing L-shape exercise 1, primarily due to stiffness in the hip joints and the back, which creates difficulty in stretching the legs.

1. Lie on the back, raise the knees, and pull them toward the abdomen. Ensure that the back is kept on the floor. If the knees

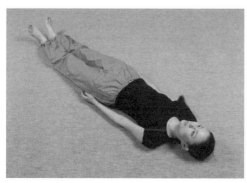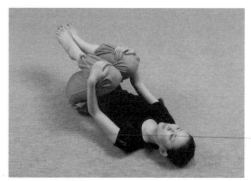

Lie on the back.

Raise the knees, and pull them toward the abdomen.

open outward in this position, it indicates a progressive stiffness in the body.

2. Spread the legs widely while keeping the knees bent.

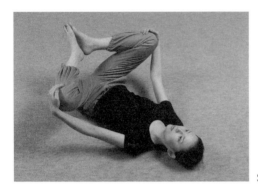

Spread the legs widely while keeping the knees bent.

3. Hold the legs wherever possible with the hands. Stretch the legs out and push the heels out toward the ceiling to stretch the Achilles tendons. Even individuals who are inflexible can stretch the legs when they are apart. Alternately push the heels further out in slow, small movements.

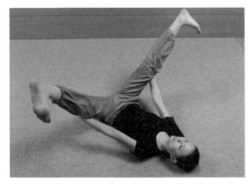

Hold the legs wherever possible with the hands.

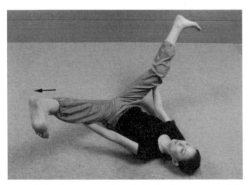 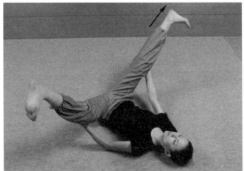

Stretch the legs out and push the heels out toward the ceiling to stretch the Achilles tendons. Alternately push the heels further out in slow, small movements.

4. Slowly bring the legs together and slowly and slighty extend the heels out further with small alternate movements, as in step 3 above. Make sure that the backs of the legs are stretched.

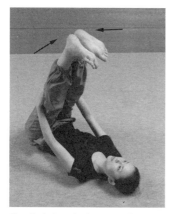
Slowly bring the legs together.

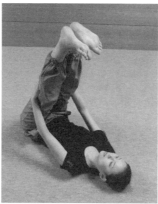
Slowly and slightly extend the heels out further with small alternate movements.

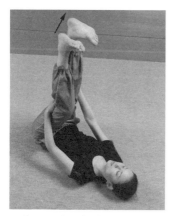
Make sure that the backs of the legs are stretched.

SACRUM EXERCISE

CAUTIONARY NOTE: Pregnant women should avoid doing this exercise.

■ EFFECTS

• Improves the symptons of the urinary organs.
• Adjusts the condition of the pelvis.

When the muscles of the lower back are tense and stiff, the lumbar spine and sacrum stiffen and cause problems in the related urinary system. For those who wake frequently during sleep because of the urge to urinate, this exercise will help to subside such urge by easing the stiffness in the lumbar and sacrum.

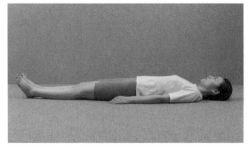

Lie on the back.

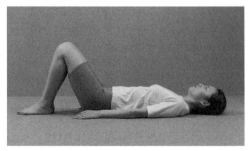

Align the heels and pull them toward the buttocks.

1. Lie on the back, align the heels, and pull them toward the buttocks.

2. Open the knees at about a 30-degree angle.

3. On exhaling, slowly lift the hips as high as possible to tighten the buttock muscles. Keep the posture for a few seconds.

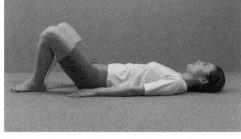

Open the knees at about a 30-degree angle.

4. On inhaling, lower the hips slowly to the floor.

Repeat the movement 2 or 3 times.

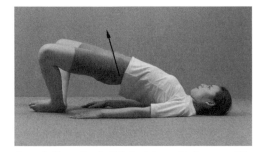

On exhaling, slowly lift the hips as high as possible to tighten the buttock muscles.

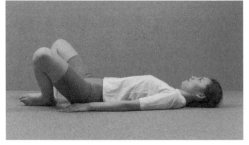

On inhaling, lower the hips slowly to the floor.

SACRUM

The sacrum is a vital area relating to various organs and systems, such as the heart, lungs, sexual organs, urinary organs, digestive organs, the nervous system, and the skin.

In the case of a burn or scald, for example, an abnormality appears in the sacrum without exception. The healing process is significantly enhanced and scarring is avoided by manipulating the abnormality.

In professional Seitai treatment, manipulation of the sacrum is used to lead the body toward a fundamental improvement in constitution, to maintain favorable changes in the body.

It is highly effective to apply DOU-KI to the sacrum as treatment for diseases in the areas mentioned above.

PUBIC BONE EXERCISE

CAUTIONARY NOTE: Pregnant women should avoid doing this exercise.

■ EFFECTS

• Improves the symptoms of gynecological disorders.
• Adjusts the pelvis after childbirth.

This exercise concentrates strength into the pubic bone using the movement of the pelvis and shoulder blades. The exercise is designed to adjust pelvic deformation and to bring the shoulder blades that have shifted laterally outward back toward the central vertical axis and their normal position.

1. Sit on the floor with the legs stretched forward. Spread the legs as wide as possible, supporting the upper body with the arms.

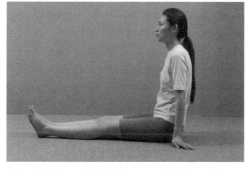

Sit on the floor with the legs stretched forward.

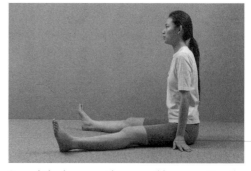

Spread the legs as wide as possible, supporting the upper body with the arms.

2. Lift the knees and pull the feet toward the buttocks, keeping the legs apart. Support the upper body by positioning the arms and hands directly under the shoulders.

3. Alternately rotate each arm backward, making sure that the chest opens and the shoulder blade slides toward the center.

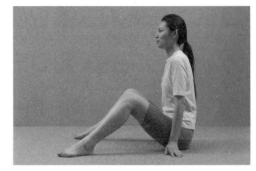

Lift the knees and pull the feet toward the buttocks, keeping the legs apart.

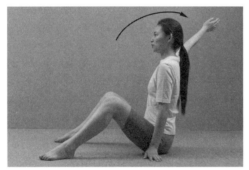 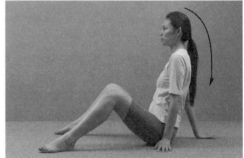

Alternately rotate the each arm backward.

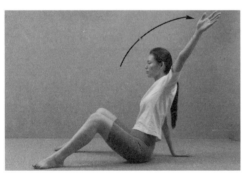 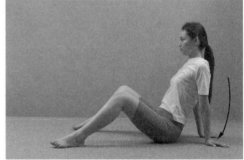

Make sure that the chest opens and the shoulder blade slides toward the center. Position the body once both arms have been rotated.

4. Position the body as shown in the picture once both arms have been rotated.

5. With the feet turned inward, lift and arch the back. Tighten the knees together while raising the hips and back.

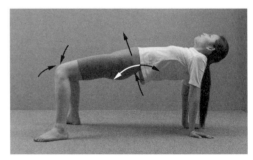

With the feet turned inward, lift and arch the back.

6. When holding the position as shown in the picture, push the pubic bone obliquely upward while further tightening the knees.

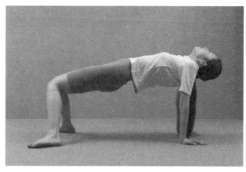

Push the pubic bone obliquely upward while further tightening the knees.

7. Slide the shoulder blades further toward the center while slowly shifting the center of gravity toward the arms.

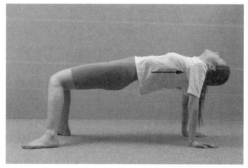

Slide the shoulder blades further toward the center.

8. Slowly shift the center of gravity toward the legs. When the position is reached where maximum strength is felt in the pelvis, hold the position for 2–3 breaths, and lower the back to the floor.

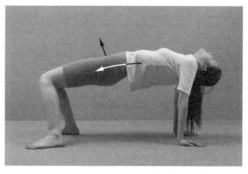

Slowly shift the center of gravity toward the legs.

C-SHAPE EXERCISE

In this exercise, a C-shape is formed by the body. Difficulty or pain encountered when stretching indicates problematic areas of the body.

1. Lie on the back. Grasp the left wrist with the right hand. Stretch the arms lightly.

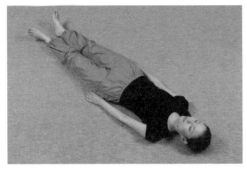
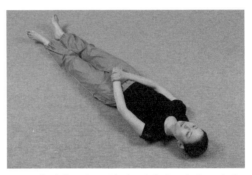

Lie on the back.

Grasp the left wrist with the right hand. Stretch the arms lightly.

2. Slowly raise the stretched arms out and up over the head.

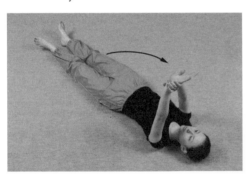
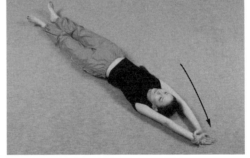

Slowly raise the stretched arms out and up over the head.

3. Stretch the arms upward and legs downward. Push the heels out to stretch the backs of the legs.

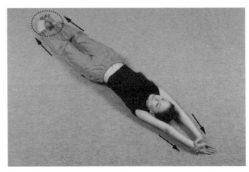

Stretch the arms upward and legs downward. Push the heels out to stretch the backs of the legs. Cross the feet inward and tightly cross the toes.

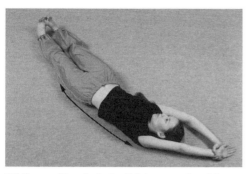

While stretching the body slightly upward and downward, slowly incline toward the right side.

4. Cross the feet inward and tightly cross the toes while stretching the legs.

5. While stretching the body slightly upward and downward, slowly incline toward the right side so as to form a 'C' with the rib area and side of the body. Incline to the furthest angle possible and hold the position.

6. Holding the angled position, again stretch the arms upward and legs downward as much as possible. Hold the position for 2–3 breaths and release the tension.

✕

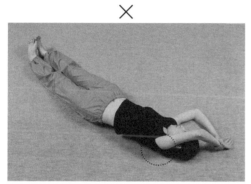

Do not lift the shoulder and the arms from the floor.

Pain or difficulty felt somewhere during the stretch indicates a problem in that area.

(a) When an abnormality is felt in a localized area: release the tension slowly while exhaling.

(b) When an abnormality is felt across a wide area: release the tension fully at one time in order to create the largest impact on the wider area.

Experiencing difficulty forming a C-shape with the body may indicate stiffness in the entire body, or in the spinal column and/or ribs.

NOTE: This exercise will not be effective if the back or shoulders are forcibly raised off the floor while trying to incline the body.

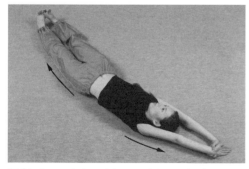

Hold the angled position, again stretch the arms upward and legs downward as much as possible.

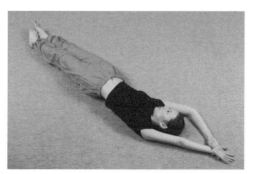

Hold the position for 2–3 breaths and release the tension.

SEITAI FIRST AID METHODS

Seitai offers many simple yet effective first aid methods to treat various symptoms. The following are two exemplary methods:

1. Anti-Suppuration Point (ASP) —*Kano-Katten*—

The anti-suppuration (to form or discharge pus) point is a vital point at the base of the deltoid muscle in the arm. The point is used to stop blood flow and suppuration related to an external injury. Stimulating the ASP activates lymph function, which protects the body from bacterial infection and viruses, and promotes healing of injuries, including postoperative incisions. It is also effective to apply the ASP method for burns or scalds as well as after dental treatment.

When an external injury occurs, a node appears in the ASP. Pinch the point and apply DOU-KI. Use the ASP on the right arm for injuries to the right half of the body and the ASP on the left arm for injuries to the left half of the body.

In the event of an injury in the lower half of the body below the navel, pinch the node at the base of the adductor muscle on the inside of the thigh of the injured side of the body and apply DOU-KI.

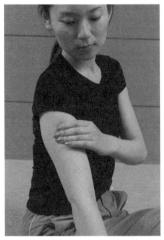

Pinch the point and apply DOU-KI. Use the ASP on the right arm for injuries in the right half of the body and the ASP on the left arm for injuries on the left half of the body.

2. Anti-Poisoning Point (APP) —*Risho-Katten*—

The anti-poisoning point is located at the junction of the right rectus abdominis muscle and the lowest right rib. Apply DOU-KI on the node located below the rib or to the inside of the ribcage. The APP is located near the liver, which works to detoxify the body. Stimulating the APP smoothly promotes the excretion of harmful substances in the case of food poisoning and acute poisoning caused by medicine. The subsequent excretion, which appears in the form of vomiting, diarrhea, or eczema, and is a normal bodily function to eliminate harmful matter from the body, requires no attention.

Chronic mental stress also appears as stiffening in the APP.

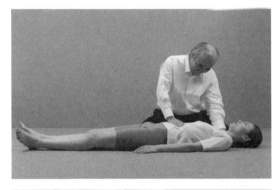

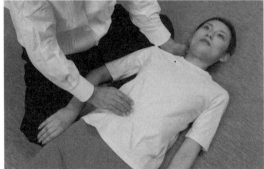

APP. Apply DOU-KI on the node located below the rib or to the inside of the ribcage.

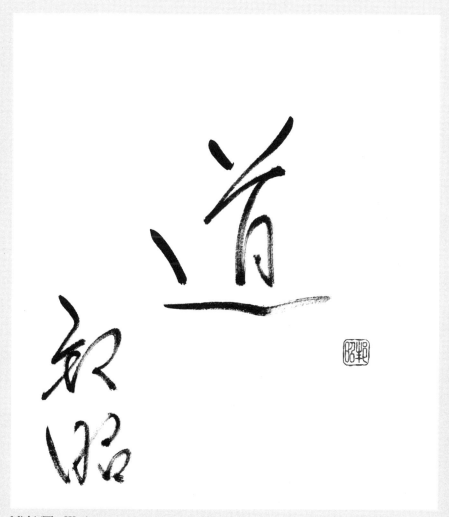

Michi (The Way)
Calligraphy by the author

SUMMARY BY SYMPTOMS

SYMPTOM	CAUSE	BODY PART	TREATMENT	HOT MOIST TOWEL TREATMENT
Headache	Problems of circulation in the entire body, especially in the upper neck	C1, C2	Recover the flexibility of the body	C1, C2 related to the medulla oblongata
Strained back	Long-term fatigue in the lumbar region	Lumbar region, mainly L1, L3, L5	Exercise for strained back; side abdomen treatment; lower back exercise	Aching part in the lumbar region
Sciatica	Long-term fatigue in the lumbar region	L4, L5	Hip joint exercise (V-shape); L-shape exercise; exercise for stiff shoulders	Base of lumbar (around L4, L5 and ilium)
Knee pain	Trouble in the lumbar region	L3	Exercise for knee pain	Aching part in the knee joint
Herniated disk	Mental stress, excessive fatigue, etc.	Mainly L4, L5	Exercise for strained back; L-shape exercise	Aching part in the lumbar region
Chronic lower back pain	Loss of flexibility in the lumbar region.	L1, L4, L5	Side abdomen treatment; deep breathing method; ilium exercise	Aching part in the lumbar region and opposing side in the abdomen
Jaw joint disorder	Mainly problems in the respiratory system	C5, C6; T3, T4	Exercise for loosening the spinal column	Part of jaw joint where aching is felt when opening the mouth.
Toothache	Fatigue, distortion of ilium	Ilium	Ilium exercise	Occipital region
Hemorrhoids	Dysfunction in the heart	T3, T4	Increase perspiration, exercise of T3&T4; ilium exercise; C shape exercise	Directly on anus
Gout	Weakening of heart, liver and kidneys; overeating	T7-T10	Foot bath; expanding the gap between the bones in the forepart of the feet	T4, T10 limited to supplementary use
Rheumatism	Dysfunction in the heart, spleen, kidneys, and liver	T4, T7-T10	Foot bath; arm bath; combined exercise; lymph exercise; C-shape exercise	Aching part
Stomach cramp	Mental stress, overeating	T6, T7, T8	DOU-KI; tightening up the ribs	Pit of stomach
Stiff shoulders	Distortion of lumbar region	Mainly C7; T1-4, T6; L2, L3	SANRI; exercise for stiff shoulders	Aching part in the shoulder
Shoulder pain caused by aging	Downward shift of pelvis due to aging	C7, T1, T3, T4, T6-8	Hot bath; breast bone exercise; exercise for stiff shoulders	Aching part in the shoulder
Shoulder joint pain	Poor circulation	C7, T1, T4	Shoulder joint exercise	Aching part in the shoulder
Other shoulder joint pain	Problems in the lungs, overuse of the arms	C7, T1, T3, T4	Exercise for stiff shoulders; breastbone exercise; exercise for shoulder joint	Aching part in the shoulder
Eye strain	Mental fatigue	C1-3	Sufficient rest of the eyes; exercise of the eyes; DOU-KI on the eyes	Around closed eyes, including temples
Dry eye	Poor perspiration, decline of function of sphincter controlling secretion of tears	T4, T5	Increase perspiration; DOU-KI	On closed eyes
Insomnia	Lack of fatigue or excessive fatigue		Exercise for pectoralis major muscles; exercise to raise the ribs; DOU-KI	Upper chest
Stiff neck after sleep	Fatigue of digestive organs	T6, T7; C7	Combined exercise; stretch and twist exercise	On the neck after Seitai exercise
Diarrhea	Natural reaction of the body to excrete unnecessary or harmful elements; sometimes hypersensitivity		Exercise for loosening spinal column; leg bath	Lower abdomen
Athlete's foot	Deterioration of blood and lymph circulation	T4	Drying the affected part with hair dryer; expanding the gap between the bones in the forepart of the feet; C-shape exercise	

SYMPTOM	CAUSE	BODY PART	TREATMENT	HOT MOIST TOWEL TREATMENT
Mental stress	Stiffness in the body	T3, T4	Rotating thumbs and big toes; exercise for loosening the spinal column; deep breathing method	Chest/pit of stomach
Swelling of foot	Decline of function of heart, kidneys and liver; fatigue	T3, T4, T9,T10	Exercise for relaxing ankles; foot bath; L-shape exercise	
Common cold	Natural reaction of the body to recover its balance	Individual part accumulating fatigue	Partial bath; individual exercise for partial fatigue	Upper neck to draw fever
Pollinosis	Stiffness of the body	Entire body, especially the thorax (chest)	Exercise for loosening spinal column; lymph exercise; breastbone exercise	Upper neck for easing runny nose and sneezes
Energy loss	Mental stress	T3, T4; L4, L5; S2	Exercise for loosening spinal column; ilium exercise; hip joint exercise	On the chest to temporarily ease mental stress
Poor complexion	Poor circulation	T3, T4	Exercise for loosening spinal column; lymph exercise; C-shape exercise	Hands and legs; part where the obstruction is felt in C-shape exercise
Heart palpitations	Excessive burden on the heart	T3, T4; L4	C-shape exercise	Center of the chest
High blood pressure	Contraction of thorax; arteriosclerosis	T8	combined exercise; lymph exercise	T8
Indigestion	Overeating, mental stress	T10–12	Lessen food intake; combined exercise	Pit of stomach
Pseudo myopia	Distortion of pelvis	Pelvis; C1–3	Ilium exercise; L-shape exercise; lift up occipital region	On closed eyes
Chronic fatigue	Stiffness of the body	Entire body	Deep breathing method	Lumbar region; lower abdomen
Constipation	Overeating	T6, T10, T11; L2	Lessen food intake; exercise for overeating; exercise for constipation	Lower abdomen
Obesity	Distortion of ilium	Ilium	Ilium exercise; breastbone exercise; pubic bone exercise; pelvis exercise	
Cystitis	Excessive fatigue	T4, T5, T10; L3, L5	Exercise for L5	Lower abdomen
Menstrual pain	Flexibility of pelvis	L4	Foot bath; ilium exercise; pubic bone exercise; exercise for prevention of menstrual pain	L4/Lower abdomen
Gallstones	Mental stress; insufficient sleep	T9	Combined exercise	Pit of stomach
Menopausal disorders	Body stiffness	L4	Exercise for loosening spinal column	Chest
Sensitivity to cold	Body stiffness; weak function of the heart and lungs; poor perspiration	T4, T5	Increase perspiration; foot bath; breastbone exercise	
Tonsillitis	Dysfunction of kidneys	C5, C6; T5, T10; L3	Footbath	On the aching part of throat to ease acute pain
Tympanitis	Overeating	C4; T5, T6	Exercise for loosening spinal column; combined exercise	Ears
Asthma	Mental Complex; naturally weak respiratory system; overeating	T3, T4	Increase perspiration; C-shape exercise; breastbone exercise; lymph exercise	Throat and upper chest
Atopic dermatitis	Lungs; maladjustment to environmental circumstances due to body stiffness	T3, T4	Breastbone exercise; deep breathing method	Inflamed areas

(英文版) 井本整体

The Seitai Method

2004 年 12 月15日　第 1 刷発行

著　者　　井本邦昭
訳　者　　ウィリアム・フェドチャック、嶋峰 誠
発行者　　畑野文夫
発行所　　講談社インターナショナル株式会社
　　　　　〒112-8652 東京都文京区音羽 1-17-14
　　　　　電話　03-3944-6493（編集部）
　　　　　　　　03-3944-6492（営業部・業務部）
　　　　　ホームページ　www.kodansha-intl.com
印刷・製本所　大日本印刷株式会社